Cholesterol
Check

Cholesterol Check

Dr Alan Maryon Davis

BBC BOOKS

Published by BBC Books,
a division of BBC Enterprises Limited,
Woodlands, 80 Wood Lane, London W12 0TT

First published 1991

ISBN 0 563 36303 7

Illustrations by Eugene Fleury

Set in Itek Galliard by Ace Filmsetting Ltd, Frome

Printed and bound in Great Britain by Clays Ltd, St Ives Plc
Cover printed by Clays Ltd, St Ives Plc

This book accompanies the series *Health UK Cholesterol Check*, made by
Prospect Pictures for BBC Wales and Daytime UK. The series was first
broadcast on BBC1 in the autumn of 1991.

Contents

About the Author

Dr Alan Maryon Davis is familiar to millions as a writer and broadcaster on health issues. He is a regular columnist for *Woman* magazine, has written several books on medical subjects ranging from the joys and perils of drink to basic first aid, has a weekly slot on LBC radio in London, and was, for many years, co-presenter of the popular BBC TV series *Bodymatters*. In his 'spare' time he is a consultant and senior lecturer in public health medicine, and lives with his wife and two daughters in South London. He lists his recreations as 'eating well, drinking well, and singing (not-so-well) with the humorous group Instant Sunshine'.

Acknowledgements

I would especially like to thank Anne Heughan of the Coronary Prevention Group, whose advice was always most timely and helpful, particularly with regard to the Mediterranean diet. Thanks also to Jennifer Jones and Tessa Clark of BBC Books, who were unfalteringly supportive and skilful as editors. And much gratitude to my dear friend Tony McAvoy of Prospect Pictures for masterminding the BBC *Health UK* series and persuading me to become so closely involved.

Why All the Fuss?

Perhaps you've seen something about it on television, heard it mentioned on radio, or come across it in a magazine – and you want to find out more.

Perhaps you've been told by your doctor that you've got rather too much of it in your bloodstream – and you feel you should do something about it.

Or perhaps you know that it's a major cause of the biggest killer disease of the Western world – coronary heart disease – and you need practical guidance on how you and your family can do your best to keep it under control.

The coronary epidemic
Whatever your reason for being interested in cholesterol, it gives rise to a great deal of concern among doctors, and other health experts, particularly in developed countries.

Britain, for example, is still in the midst of what has been described as an 'epidemic' of premature coronary heart disease, with one of the world's highest death rates: four out of every 10 men who die in middle age. Other countries in northern and eastern Europe, North America, Australia and New Zealand have suffered similarly.

A key factor
We now know that one of the key reasons why so many people in Western countries die young from a heart attack is because most of us have too much cholesterol in our

bloodstream. A high blood cholesterol multiplies the dangers of a whole string of other factors – being overweight, lack of exercise, smoking, stress, high blood pressure, diabetes and family heart trouble. All these work together to push up our risk of falling victim to a heart attack, angina or that other disorder caused by diseased arteries – a stroke.

Of course, within each and every one of us there are other factors, which we don't yet understand so well, that ultimately determine how important a part our blood cholesterol will actually play in our future health. But there's no doubt that keeping cholesterol under control could make all the difference between life and death for a great many of us.

And there's equally no doubt that the single most important way in which most of us can control our cholesterol is by eating less fatty food and more cereals, vegetables and fruit.

Clearing up the confusion

Despite the worldwide mountain of evidence for this, you'll still hear claims that the scientists have got it all wrong, that there's nothing harmful in the average person's diet, that fat is beautiful, that exercise is a killer and that heart disease is anyway the best way to go.

You'll also hear that the real answer to cholesterol is this or that wonder cure: garlic, oatbran, nicotinic acid, lecithin, fish oil or simply half an aspirin a day.

No wonder so many people are confused and worried.

Later on in this book we'll sift through the evidence, and help you sort fact from fantasy.

Making changes

Our main purpose is to show how you can make a few changes to bring down the overall risk for yourself and your family.

We'll show you how to choose and prepare a healthy balance of delicious food to help you keep your cholesterol, and your weight, nicely down.

We'll describe how exercise can improve your blood-fat profile as well as your body shape.

We'll help you overcome the ravages of stress, and give guidance on how to stop smoking and cut down on your drinking.

And we'll look at what's involved in having a check-up for blood cholesterol and blood pressure, and how medical treatment can bring improvement when natural self-help methods are not quite enough.

Start now

There's firm evidence that all these factors can begin to affect our arteries surprisingly early in life, perhaps even in childhood. All the more reason, therefore, if you have a young family, to start putting this good advice into practice right now.

Even if you're beyond this stage, and want to give your heart a better chance in the second half of your life, it's not too late. You can still do a lot to reduce your risks and make a brand-new start in life.

– 1 –
Heart Disease and Strokes: the Basic Facts

Few illnesses can be more sudden, or more potentially disastrous, than either a heart attack or a stroke.

Both happen like a bolt from the blue, often without warning. One minute everything's fine, the next minute someone's life is in grave danger.

With a heart attack, part of the heart muscle is damaged, threatening to weaken the heartbeat or stop it altogether.

With a stroke, the damage is to part of the brain, causing paralysis, numbness or some other impairment – often permanently.

Yet, although very different from each other, these two dreadful disorders have a common root cause: the arterial disease, atherosclerosis.

And although each tragedy may be sudden and unheralded, the underlying disease has been building up slowly and insidiously for decades.

In this chapter, we look at the basics of heart disease and strokes. What symptoms do they cause? What actually goes wrong? What exactly is atherosclerosis?

And we see how cholesterol fits into this story.

The heart of the problem
Reg, 62, is watching television – the big match. His team is about to score, and he's on the edge of his seat, punching the air and yelling at the screen.

Suddenly he starts to feel a pain across his chest – a dull, vague pain, welling up like bad indigestion. He tries belching to get rid of it – but it doesn't help. The pain worsens, like a huge weight pressing on his chest. He tries to get to his feet, but he feels faint and breaks out in a cold sweat. The pain seems to be crushing his chest and rising into his throat. He struggles for air, and calls to his wife, Jean.

She sees him looking dreadfully grey and clearly in great pain. It takes her a while to find out what's happening. She settles Reg back in the chair, and gets him a brandy to sip. Her immediate thought is that he might be having a heart attack. Reg says not to bother the doctor – but Jean rings up anyway.

Margaret, 54, has been feeling more and more tired these last few months, which she puts down to being 19 kg (3 stones) overweight.

About 4 weeks ago, she had to break into a bit of a run to catch the bus into town, and as she pulled herself on board she felt a terrible tight pain in her chest, which took quite a few minutes to ease off. She thought perhaps she'd strained a muscle.

Now this past fortnight, she's had the same pain several times, especially when she's climbing stairs or walking up the hill to the corner shop. It's a nasty, heavy, dull pain, which stops her in her tracks – and then eases off after she's rested for a minute or two.

But it's beginning to bother her – so she makes up her mind to see the doctor about it.

Harry, 58, looks anxiously at his watch. Four minutes to nine. Yet again the train has let him down – him and everyone else in the crammed carriage. At last it pulls into the station, and the hordes pour out. Harry hurries towards the ticket barrier to avoid the usual bottleneck, but he is hampered by all the extra documents in his briefcase. Mustn't be late . . . must press on . . .

Harry staggers and collapses unconscious before he can reach one of the platform seats, landing in a crumpled heap – his umbrella clattering under the feet of passers-by. Someone stops to help him. Another person goes to fetch the guard.

Harry is turning blue. A fellow commuter gives him mouth-to-mouth resuscitation and cardiac massage for 20 minutes before the ambulance arrives.

By the time he reaches hospital, Harry is dead.

These three case histories illustrate the three main ways in which heart disease usually becomes apparent.

Reg: heart attack

This is the classic heart attack – acute myocardial infarction or coronary thrombosis – a 'coronary' for short. The key symptom is a heavy, crushing pain, felt across the chest, perhaps radiating up to the jaw, into one or both shoulders, or even down one or both arms, most often the left. Usually the sufferer feels sweaty, faint and nauseated, and almost always has an overwhelming feeling of leaden tiredness. The pain is not quickly relieved by rest and reassurance, but takes hours to wear off.

Some heart attacks are much milder than this – and often confused with a touch of indigestion. According to ECG (electrocardiogram) traces taken at routine medical checks, many people have had a heart attack without ever realising it.

Nevertheless, any heart attack, however mild, is potentially life-threatening, and all too often heralds a further attack, perhaps more massive than before.

Margaret: angina

The second story is a typical case of angina: recurring chest pain felt on exertion, excitement or emotion, which eases off after a few minutes of rest or relaxation. Again, the pain may not be as severe as this in every case, or may be far worse. It can stay about the same for years, or it can rapidly deteriorate in a matter of days. A few very severely affected people have angina most of the time, even at rest.

Angina is the heart crying for help, as we'll see below, and it often precedes a heart attack.

Harry: sudden cardiac death

The third case history is fortunately not so common. In this case, the victim's heart suddenly stops beating (cardiac arrest), usually because the heart muscle goes into a quivering, useless state – ventricular fibrillation.

The person will die within 3 or 4 minutes unless an adequate circulation can be restored, by chest compressions (cardiac massage) or by restoring the normal heartbeat using a special electric shock machine – a defibrillator.

About four out of five people who fall victim to sudden cardiac death have a known history of heart disease, with previous angina or heart attack.

These then are the main ways heart disease can strike. But what actually goes wrong within the heart?

Heart disease – the inside story

When we talk of heart disease in relation to cholesterol, the type of 'heart disease' we are referring to is coronary heart disease – disease of the coronary arteries in the heart – which is the cause of heart attacks, angina or sudden death. Other types, such as congenital malformations or rheumatic valve disease, are much less common.

Coronary heart disease is sometimes also called 'ischaemic' heart disease. *Ischaemia* is Greek for lack of blood, and it neatly describes the underlying fault. Although the heart is full of blood, its own tissue (the heart muscle) doesn't get enough – a tragic irony if ever there was one.

Pumping power

Your heart is a fist-sized pump, its four chambers filling with blood at each beat, with flap-valves controlling the flow so that the blood enters from the main veins and is forcefully ejected into the main arteries. The pumping power comes from the muscular walls of the chambers, especially the thick-walled ventricles, whose job is to apply the necessary pressure to force the blood around the circulation. The right ventricle pumps blood through the lungs to pick up oxygen and get rid of carbon dioxide. The left ventricle, the most muscular chamber of all, pumps blood round the rest of the body.

Very special muscle

The heart muscle is quite remarkable: it pumps away, beating about 70 times a minute, non-stop for life. No other muscle in the body could keep up this kind of work for more than a few hours at a time, without seizing up with fatigue and cramp – even in the most highly trained marathon runner. But the heart muscle is specially adapted to the task and never seems to tire.

The coronary arteries

Any hard-working muscle has to have plenty of oxygen to fire its energy system, and a rapid means of removing spent fuel. The crucial requirement is a rich blood supply to do both jobs. So all rapidly contracting muscles have a very dense network of blood vessels. This is one reason why flesh is so red.

No muscle has a greater need for a thoroughly effective blood supply than the heart muscle itself. To ensure this, it receives freshly oxygenated blood through its own private arteries – the coronary arteries – which are the first branches off the aorta, the main artery.

The coronary arteries, about as wide as a drinking straw, encircle the top of the heart (*corona* is Latin for crown), before branching into smaller vessels that course all over its surface and plunge deep into its muscle, branching again and again until every part of the heart is supplied.

Because the heart has to cope with such varying demands – working up to 20 times as hard when you're exercising as when you're at rest – the coronary arteries are able to become much wider in order to carry any extra blood needed. Young people's coronary arteries can do this much more effectively than older people's. In middle age, the arterial walls begin to stiffen and they lose their elasticity (like so many other parts of the body!).

This can have important consequences if the arteries also happen to be 'furring up' inside.

Furring up

If a coronary artery, or major branch, becomes so narrowed or clogged that part of the heart is deprived of an adequate blood supply, the person will feel the characteristic heavy cardiac pain in their chest. This usually first becomes apparent during heavy exertion, or at times of excitement or emotion, when the heart is beating faster and needs more oxygen. These are the classic times for angina to strike.

If a clot, or thrombus, forms in a furred-up coronary

artery, or its branch, it can fairly rapidly narrow the blood flow still more, bringing on worsening angina (sometimes called 'crescendo angina').

If the clot builds up so rapidly that it completely blocks the artery (coronary thrombosis) the part of the heart muscle supplied by that blood vessel is suddenly deprived of all its sustenance. The affected area gives rise to severe cardiac pain, swells a little, and soon ceases to beat with the rest of the heart. Unless the clot can be removed within an hour or so, that area of heart muscle will die (myocardial infarction).

The effect of all this will depend on how much muscle has been damaged, and whether it includes any part of the heart's internal co-ordinating system. The bigger the area of damage, the greater the risk of the heart not being able to pump effectively. And if the co-ordinating system has been hit, there's a high risk of disrupting the heart's normal rhythm – perhaps leading to the fatal complication, ventricular fibrillation.

Sometimes this happens without thrombosis – and is simply due to severe furring up of the artery supplying the system that co-ordinates heartbeats. A little extra exertion, excitement or emotion is all it may take to exceed the available blood supply and trigger the heart into ventricular fibrillation – causing cardiac arrest and sudden death.

What is a stroke?
People sometimes get confused between a heart attack and a stroke. The two names have a similar ring, and both disorders are sudden catastrophes with potentially dire consequences. Just to add to the confusion, a stroke can sometimes follow close on the heels of a heart attack.

But with a stroke, the seat of the damage is the brain rather than the heart.

It's more difficult to describe a typical stroke than a typical heart attack because strokes vary widely, depending on which part of the brain is affected and how badly. But a very common form is one in which the major part of one cerebral hemisphere is put out of action, resulting in weakness or paralysis down the whole of the opposite side of the body – hemiplegia. If, as usually happens, the sensory area of the hemisphere is also affected there will be loss of feeling in addition to the weakness. And if the affected hemisphere is the 'dominant' one (usually the left hemisphere) speech is likely to be disrupted.

The damage to the brain is caused in one of three ways.

The commonest cause, accounting for about half of all strokes, is cerebral thrombosis, in which an artery to the brain becomes blocked with a developing clot. Brain tissue is extremely sensitive to a lack of oxygen and, with its blood supply cut off, the area of brain supplied by the blocked artery ceases to function and is irreversibly damaged within a few minutes.

Another common cause, accounting for about one stroke in three, is cerebral embolism, in which an obstruction, usually a loose clot, is swept up in the bloodstream to the brain and gets stuck in one of its branching arteries, causing a blockage. The effects are indistinguishable from those caused by thrombosis. The source of the loose clot in many cases is the heart – particularly in people recovering from a recent heart attack – a cruel double blow.

The third, and least common, cause of a stroke is cerebral haemorrhage, in which an artery coursing over or through the brain ruptures and bleeds, pressing on the neighbouring brain tissue. The effects of this will depend very much on how much bleeding has occurred, and which part of the brain has been damaged.

Strokes are unlikely under the age of about 60 – but the risk increases rapidly after that, as the arteries lose more and more of their strength and elasticity. Added to this normal ageing effect are the consequences of two further risk factors: high blood pressure and atherosclerosis.

High blood pressure increases the risk of cerebral thrombosis or haemorrhage by straining the arteries, which weakens them further, and also by subjecting the blood flow to extra turbulence.

Atherosclerosis furs up the arteries with fatty deposits which may either lead to cerebral thrombosis, by acting as a focus for the sudden formation of a blood clot, or may slowly restrict the blood supply to various parts of the brain causing intermittent bouts of giddiness, weakness, numbness or pins and needles, known as transient ischaemic attacks.

Atherosclerosis: your arteries' arch-enemy

Vital pipes

Your arteries are the vital pipes which convey bright red oxygenated blood, under pressure, from your heart to all parts of your body, dividing into smaller and smaller branches until eventually they reach the network of microscopic capillaries weaving through the tissues.

There, the blood gives up its oxygen and nutrients and picks up carbon dioxide and other waste products, becoming a dark magenta colour. Then it seeps into tiny venules, the tributaries of larger and larger veins, and flows sluggishly back to the heart.

Because the blood in your arteries is under pressure, fluctuating with each beat of your heart, the arterial walls have to be tough but elastic, rather like a rubber hose, stretching a little as each pulse-wave passes through and bouncing back immediately afterwards. And to ensure that the flow of blood is as smooth as possible, with a minimum

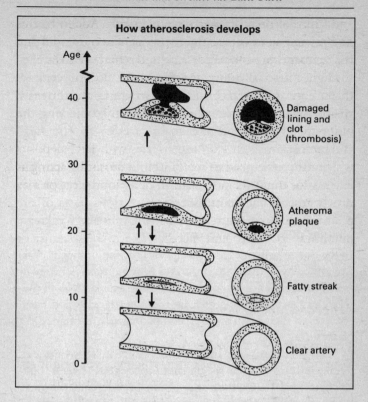

How atherosclerosis develops

Age

40 —

30 —

20 —

10 —

0 —

Damaged lining and clot (thrombosis)

Atheroma plaque

Fatty streak

Clear artery

of friction, the inner linings of the arteries have to be ultra-sleek and squeaky clean.

This is how your arteries started out in your youth – supple and smooth-bored. The chances are they haven't stayed that way. They are almost certainly succumbing slowly to the insidious arterial disease, atherosclerosis.

Fatty deposits

Atherosclerosis is the gradual laying down of fatty deposits in the lining of arteries, which slowly form whitish, stiff, ragged patches – atheroma plaques (*athere* means porridge, and *skleros* hard, in Greek). So atherosclerosis is a form of hardening of the arteries.

Each atheroma plaque consists mainly of cholesterol and related substances, together with some calcium and the remnants of broken-down cells, covered with a layer of thickened arterial lining and fibrous tissue. The arteries that are most likely to be affected are the aorta (the main artery down the trunk), the main arteries to the legs, the coronary arteries and the main arteries to the head and brain.

The atheroma plaques steadily build up, rather like 'fur' in a kettle, gradually narrowing the bore of the arteries – a process that usually takes decades.

When does atherosclerosis begin?

One of the first clues as to when this furring up begins was provided by studying the reports of post-mortems performed on young American soldiers killed in the Korean War in the 1950s. Doctors were struck by the number who had fatty streaks in their main arteries, and particularly in their coronary arteries.

Ten years later, the International Atherosclerosis Project collected post-mortem specimens of arteries from over 22 000 people aged 10–69, both sexes, from 14 different countries. Again, extensive fatty streaks were found in a high proportion of teenagers, and quite a few children.

Although there's some dispute among the experts as to whether these fatty streaks inevitably become atheroma plaques in later life, the prevailing view is that they do represent the first stage of the atherosclerosis process.

But atheroma can develop much faster than this. Post-mortems performed on people who have died within a few years of having a coronary artery bypass graft operation have revealed many cases in which the new graft (usually a short length of leg vein) has become almost as clogged with atheroma as the original artery. This rapid re-furring usually happens only to people who have inherited a tendency to severe atherosclerosis.

It is this narrowing, and roughening of the normally silky smooth arterial lining, that can set off a train of events spelling disaster for the heart, brain or other vital organs.

Slow clogging

Firstly, as the atheroma slowly clogs an artery, the organ or tissue whose blood was being supplied by that artery becomes more and more starved of oxygen and nutrients. The effects of this lack of blood, or ischaemia, depend on which organ or tissue is affected and how much blood is managing to get through.

For example, if it's the heart the first symptom is usually angina – a heavy crushing pain in the chest, and perhaps the jaw, shoulders and left arm, not unlike the pain felt during a heart attack. It starts to come on during heavy exertion, excitement or emotion, and, unlike the heart-attack pain, eases off again with rest or relaxation. As the narrowing worsens, the angina becomes ever more severe, with less and less exertion, until eventually the sufferer may have crippling pain even at rest.

If an artery to the brain becomes gradually narrowed, the person may suffer increasingly frequent giddy spells, a poor memory or a gradual loss of intellect.

Sudden blockage

The other all-too-common consequence of atheroma plaques, and one which can strike suddenly without warning, is thrombosis. This is the rapid formation of a clot, usually where an atheroma plaque has damaged the arterial lining.

If this happens in a coronary artery or one of its branches (coronary thrombosis), the result is usually a heart attack – acute myocardial infarction.

If it happens in an artery supplying the brain, the resulting cerebral thrombosis causes a stroke.

– 2 –
What Exactly Is Cholesterol?

Friend or foe?
They say it helps to know your enemy. So what exactly is this dreaded substance that can cause so much damage?

Perhaps the first surprise is that, far from being some alien chemical, cholesterol plays a vital part in every cell of the body. It's a natural product of all animal cells, including human ones, and is a key component of cell membranes, helping to regulate what goes in and out of the cell. Without cholesterol, neither we, nor any other animal, could exist. Yet, interestingly, plants have evolved a different cell-membrane system and can manage perfectly well without it.

Another important fact is that about two-thirds of the cholesterol in the body is synthesised in the liver from substances derived from the fat in our food, and that this process is closely controlled. The rest comes mainly via the wall of the small intestine, where it's partly synthesised from fats in the diet, and partly absorbed directly from the cholesterol we eat.

Much of our body's cholesterol is used to make bile (*chole* in Greek), the greenish liquid stored in the gall bladder, which helps to digest fatty food. Cholesterol is also used as a building block for the body's production of steroid hormones. And, last but not least as far as this book is concerned, cholesterol may also have a role as a waterproofing agent in the linings of arteries.

Candle-grease

Cholesterol is not a fat, but is a soft, waxy, fat-like substance, with the consistency of warm candle-grease. However, this is not the form in which it's transported about the body. The fluid within cells (intracellular fluid), the fluid that bathes cells (tissue fluid) and the fluid that does most of the transporting (blood) are all water-based media, and can only deal easily with water-soluble substances. Anything really fatty would just separate into greasy globules – rather like oil separating from vinegar in French dressing – clogging up all sorts of vital processes.

Tiny parcels

So how does fatty cholesterol get about? The answer is that as soon as it's made it becomes wrapped with special proteins (apoproteins) which act as a wetting agent, in effect making it water-soluble so that it can be transported, in minute 'parcels', in the body fluids and put to use where it's needed. To some extent, this is rather like the action of washing-up liquid lifting grease off the dinner dishes.

Various other fat-like substances have to be treated in a similar way. The general term for all these fatty substances, including cholesterol, is lipids (Greek again – *lipos* means fat). The tiny parcels of lipid and protein are called 'lipoproteins'. If lipid levels are too high, this is called 'hyperlipidaemia'.

Cholesterol in the blood

Cholesterol can only cause heart disease or stroke if there's too much of it in the bloodstream for too long a period. Since blood is the main vehicle for ferrying cholesterol around the body, let's take a closer look at it.

In every microscopic cubic millimetre of blood there are

about 5 500 000 red blood cells (oxygen carriers), about 10 000 white blood cells (infection fighters, antibody makers and scavengers) and about 500 000 platelets (leak sealers and clotters). This regular army is floating in plasma, a rich, slightly cloudy broth of hundreds of different substances, some dissolved, others suspended. Among the latter are the millions of lipoprotein particles containing cholesterol and other lipids. As we'll see later, the total level of cholesterol in a person's plasma (the total cholesterol or TC level) is clearly linked to their risk of developing atherosclerosis, and hence heart disease or stroke.

LDL vs HDL

There are two main types of cholesterol-carrying lipoproteins: low density and high density. About two-thirds of the cholesterol in the blood is carried in low-density lipoprotein (LDL), and most of the rest in high-density lipoprotein (HDL).

This is an important distinction. Recent evidence suggests that LDL's main job is to pick up cholesterol from the liver and distribute it around the body, including the lining of the arteries. Problems arise when too much cholesterol enters the lining, furring up the arteries.

By contrast, HDL's main task seems to be the very opposite. It is thought to carry cholesterol *away* from the tissues, including the arteries, and back to the liver for re-processing or breakdown.

The dynamic duo

So it looks as though the two main types of lipoprotein act as a duo, adjusting the supply of cholesterol to and from the liver and maintaining a balance. If indeed this were so, it would be an important control mechanism and you might expect the balance of LDL to HDL to have a bearing on a person's risk of atherosclerosis: the higher their LDL (cholesterol on its way to the arterial lining and elsewhere), the higher their risk – and the higher the HDL (cholesterol being removed from the arterial lining and elsewhere), the *lower* their risk.

In other words, HDL could have a 'protective' effect.

Triglycerides

As if things weren't complicated enough, here's yet another chemical term you may hear bandied about: 'triglycerides', a family of related substances. But don't be confused by the jargon. They are simply common-or-garden fats. Nearly all the fat and oil we eat is in the form of triglycerides. Lard is a mixture of different ones. So too is butter, margarine, olive oil, sunflower oil . . . For 'triglycerides' simply read 'fat'.

The fat in our food is digested by enzymes and absorbed by the small intestine. Microscopic globules, together with a little cholesterol, are then wrapped in a thin lipoprotein coat and passed into the bloodstream. These micro-bubbles are called 'chylomicrons', and are about one-eighth of the diameter of a red blood cell.

Milky plasma

After any meal containing fat or oil, your plasma becomes quite milky with chylomicrons as they make their way from the small intestine to the fat-storage tissues: adipose tissue (body fat) and muscles. Within a few hours, their contents have been stored away, their remnants have been re-processed by the liver, and once again, the plasma becomes relatively clear.

Because chylomicrons contain some cholesterol along

with the triglycerides, they raise the total level of blood cholesterol whenever they're present in the bloodstream. If a sample of your blood is taken within a few hours of a meal your total cholesterol level will therefore be higher than usual, distorting your blood-lipid profile to some extent. You may be asked to avoid food for several hours beforehand, to provide a 'fasting' cholesterol level.

Your blood-lipid profile

We've now looked at cholesterol – where it comes from, where it goes to and how it gets there. Let's summarise the main points:

✳ Cholesterol is a natural substance, vital to every cell in the body. It is also used to make bile, various hormones and other important organic chemicals.

✳ Most of your cholesterol (at least two-thirds) is manufactured in the liver by converting fat. Most of the rest is synthesised in the cells of the small intestine, again from fat. Only a minor proportion of your body's cholesterol is derived directly from any cholesterol in your food.

✳ Cholesterol is transported through your body in your blood plasma, in three main forms: 60–70 per cent in low-density lipoprotein (LDL); 20–30 per cent in high-density lipoprotein (HDL); and the remainder, together with triglycerides, in chylomicrons.

✳ Your total cholesterol level (TC) is the key measurement, particularly if it's your fasting level. This has a very strong bearing on your risk of furred-up arteries and hence heart disease and stroke. Broadly speaking, the higher your TC, the higher your risk.

✳ But another key measurement is your HDL. This indicates a protective effect for your arteries. The higher your HDL level, the *lower* your risk.

✳ Your blood also contains another type of lipid – triglycerides (fat) – especially after meals. Some are still present between meals, and your fasting level of triglycerides may have a bearing on your coronary risk. But this link isn't yet firmly established.

Cholesterol in your food

A word about the cholesterol in food – dietary cholesterol. It's found almost entirely with animal fats – in fatty meat and meat products, offal, egg yolks and, oddly enough, in some shellfish. The key point is that dietary cholesterol usually contributes only a small proportion of the total cholesterol in your bloodstream. In fact, the amount of *fat* you eat, especially saturated fat, is much more important as far as your blood cholesterol is concerned.

We'll be looking much more closely at the major part your diet plays in determining your cholesterol level, and hence your risk, in Chapter 5.

— 3 —
Who's Most at Risk?
And Why?

If you were asked to describe a typical heart-attack victim, the chances are you would say it's a middle-aged man, very overweight and out of condition, in a high-pressure job, who eats nothing but fried food and is a chain-smoker. You might add that his father died of a coronary at 50.

Certainly, anyone fitting this description would be a prime candidate for an early demise from heart disease. But, in fact, only a small minority of heart-attack victims match up to this identikit picture. For most, the presence of just a few of these so-called 'risk factors' is enough.

So, who is most at risk? What sort of person? And why? What kind of lifestyle do they have? And, in particular, what eating, drinking and smoking habits are most likely to add to their risk?

This chapter answers these questions – and looks at the evidence we have to back up our knowledge of the many risk factors for heart disease and strokes.

How important is your age?
It's an irrefutable fact that the older we are, the more likely we are to die from coronary heart disease or a stroke. The evidence for this comes from national mortality statistics, based on the compulsory certification of all deaths.

For example, in Western nations like the United Kingdom, men are about 15 times more likely to die from a heart attack between the ages of 55 and 64 than they are between 35 and 44. In women, the increase in risk over the same 20 years is 30-fold. And above the age of 65, the risk of having a heart attack or stroke zooms up even higher in both sexes.

But why the rapidly worsening odds as we get older? Most experts agree that it's likely to be due mainly to the accumulated effect of years of having a high blood cholesterol, high blood pressure and other factors, all increasing the risk of atherosclerosis in the arteries.

How about sex?

There's no doubt that men are more at risk of coronary heart disease and strokes than women of the same age. Again, mortality statistics provide the evidence.

With heart disease, the difference is most striking in the younger age-groups: for example, men aged 35–44 are nearly six times more likely to die of a heart attack than their female counterparts.

But this particular form of sex discrimination diminishes as we get older, so that by the time we reach about 85 the two sexes have an almost equal risk of having a heart attack – but not quite. The main change for women occurs between the ages of 45 and 54, when their risk rises quite rapidly towards that of men.

Research indicates that the reason why women seem to be partly 'protected' against heart disease under the age of about 50 is probably linked to the effect of oestrogen, the female hormone. This would explain why they seem to lose their protection when they go through the menopause – when their oestrogen level falls dramatically. Quite how oestrogen exerts this so-called 'protective' effect is not yet known.

As far as the risk of a stroke is concerned, men are only

slightly more prone than women of the same age, but this difference increases over the age of about 60, when men become much more likely than women to have a stroke. This is more difficult to explain. Although women lose their relative immunity against heart disease with the menopause, they seem to remain less vulnerable than men to strokes.

Nationality and race

No nation or race on Earth seems to be immune from the ravages of atherosclerosis or coronary heart disease. International studies show that all racial groups so far investigated are vulnerable to these disorders.

Nevertheless, some are much more vulnerable than others. There are certainly big differences in the death rates from heart disease between various countries, as you can see from the 'league table' opposite.

So why these differences? How much is due to genetic factors in the racial make-up of the different populations? And how much is linked to people's dietary habits or other aspects of their lifestyle?

An important clue comes from a study of Japanese men. In Japan, both sexes have an extremely low rate of heart disease and, as the table shows, that country is firmly at the bottom of the international heart-risk league.

But when Japanese men living in Japan were compared with racially identical men living in Hawaii, the latter were found to be much more prone to heart disease – by about half as much again. And when the comparison was made with ethnic Japanese men living in California, the prevalence of heart disease almost doubled. So it looks as though there's something about the change of environment that tends to cancel out what seems at first sight to be a natural 'immunity' to heart disease.

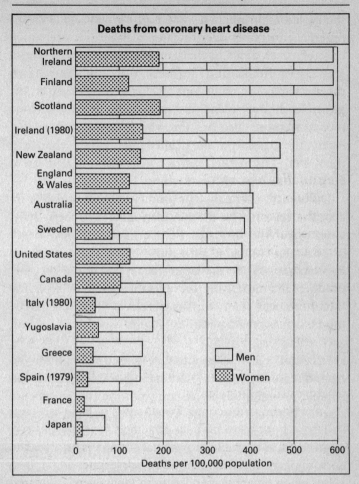

Deaths from coronary heart disease

Deaths per 100,000 population

(Men / Women by country: Northern Ireland, Finland, Scotland, Ireland (1980), New Zealand, England & Wales, Australia, Sweden, United States, Canada, Italy (1980), Yugoslavia, Greece, Spain (1979), France, Japan)

What's the most likely explanation for this? Is it because there's more stress in Hawaii or California than Japan? Hardly! Do people smoke more in America than Japan? No, that's certainly not true – and, anyway, smoking habits were taken into account in calculating the study's results.

Most experts agree that the culprit is almost certainly the change in dietary habits among those Japanese who emigrate to Hawaii and California. We certainly know that the typical Californian fast-food diet is a far cry from the traditional seafood and rice eaten in Japan!

There is a similar development among the Eskimos (Inuits) of Alaska and northern Canada. Their heart-disease rates used to be among the lowest of any ethnic group in the world, but are now rising as they become more and more absorbed into the American way of life. Again, the experts put the blame largely on the change in their diet – from the traditional fish and seal meat to burgers and chips with everything.

Differences in the type of food people eat is also probably the reason why the populations of southern Italy, Greece and the south of France have such low heart-disease rates compared with those of places like Scotland and Finland. While the latter have a diet based on dairy products and meat, with few vegetables and fresh fruit, the 'Mediterranean' diet consists largely of fibre-rich starchy food (such as bread, potatoes or pasta) and plenty of fruit and vegetables.

In Britain, racial subgroups vary in their susceptibility to heart disease and strokes. With heart disease, the most vulnerable communities are Asians from the Indian subcontinent. With strokes, Afro-Caribbeans and Africans are most at risk. Again, it looks as though these differences are partly a matter of genes and partly diet. Asians have a higher genetic tendency to have diabetes, a disorder linked to heart disease – but in addition their traditional diet includes ghee, a butter-like fat. People of African or Afro-Caribbean stock have an in-built susceptibility to high blood pressure, a well-known risk factor for heart disease and, more particularly, strokes.

So the message is clear enough. Although nationalities and some racial groups seem to have either a 'natural' resistance, or vulnerability, to heart disease or strokes – due in part to their genes – this protection or proneness

The Framingham Heart Study

Most of the evidence about heart-disease risk factors, that we now take more or less for granted, comes from an immensely painstaking research study started in the late 1940s in the small town of Framingham, situated about 29 km (18 miles) west of Boston, Massachusetts, USA. Some 5000 men and women aged 30–59 agreed to have a full health check every two years, for as long as the study lasted. The health checks were offered free of charge, so, bearing in mind the usual cost of medical care in America, perhaps it's not surprising that so many people agreed to take part. What they didn't bargain for was that the study would be running more than 35 years later!

Thanks to these obliging townsfolk of Framingham, over 3000 of whom have sadly died from various causes in the meantime, the research investigators have been able to collect a mountain of information, detailing exactly how a whole range of factors can be linked to the subsequent health and illness of the participants. We can see, for example, whether those who were overweight really were more likely to have heart attacks (they were), and whether the amount people smoked was linked to their coronary risk (it was). We can see to what extent having high blood pressure was related to the participants' risk of getting heart disease, and how those who exercised regularly were much less likely to suffer from a coronary than those who led an inactive life.

But perhaps the most striking finding from the Framingham Study was the strong link between the level of cholesterol in the participants' blood and their susceptibility to a heart attack, angina or a stroke. The message is quite clear: people with a high blood-cholesterol level are much more at risk from these disorders – and the higher the cholesterol, the higher that risk is. What's more, the Framingham Study showed that a high blood cholesterol *multiplies* the harmful effects of smoking, high blood pressure, obesity and the other risk factors.

also depends greatly on their way of life. And the one aspect of this which seems to be most influential is undoubtedly their diet.

Blood-cholesterol level

The first really convincing evidence linking cholesterol with coronary heart disease in a variety of different communities came from a pioneering research study set up in the 1950s by Professor Ancel Keys of Minneapolis, USA, together with colleagues in Japan, Yugoslavia, Finland, Italy, Greece and the Netherlands.

In this Seven Countries Study, over 12 000 men between the ages of 40 and 59 were carefully followed up for 10 years. In particular, any links between their diet, their blood-cholesterol level, and their susceptibility to coronary heart disease were noted.

The study clearly demonstrated that the average level of blood cholesterol among the men in each of the countries was strongly linked to their country's rate of coronary heart disease: the higher the blood cholesterol, the higher the risk of heart trouble. The Finnish men, for example, had far and away the highest blood-cholesterol levels, and about 13 times as many heart attacks as the Japanese!

The Seven Countries Study has been followed up by several other major pieces of research showing the link between cholesterol and heart disease – most notably, the Framingham Heart Study and the British Regional Heart Study. Both found that people with the highest levels of cholesterol had about three times the risk of heart disease than those with the lowest levels.

A particularly striking discovery came from the British study. The average middle-aged man in Britain has a blood-cholesterol level so high that it *doubles* his risk of a heart attack, compared with men of the same age with a low cholesterol level.

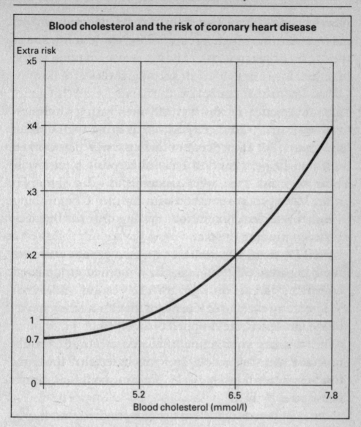

Blood cholesterol and the risk of coronary heart disease

Extra risk

Blood cholesterol (mmol/l)

Cholesterol-lowering experiments

Another way to investigate this link is to conduct an experiment by lowering people's cholesterol level and seeing how this affects their risk of getting heart disease. A group are put on a cholesterol-lowering programme – a diet plan or special drug treatment, or both – and compared with a similar group who carry on as usual.

There have been several studies trying this approach, but because atherosclerosis and heart disease take so long to develop, scientists are still waiting for clear results.

Nevertheless, there's already evidence from trials involving men with very high levels of blood cholesterol, and at therefore the greatest risk of heart disease, to point to the potential life-saving effect of keeping cholesterol down.

One impressive example is the Lipid Research Clinics Study in America, in which 18 000 men with high cholesterol levels received dietary advice to bring their cholesterol down. For 80 per cent of them the new diet worked well, but 20 per cent still had dangerously high levels. These high-risk men were randomly divided into two groups. One group carried on with the diet as before, and the other received cholesterol-lowering drug treatment as well as continuing the diet.

After 7½ years, the health of the two groups was carefully compared. Sure enough, the drug/diet group fared better than the diet-only group. Their blood-cholesterol levels were an average of 9 per cent lower, and their heart-disease incidence rate dropped by one-fifth.

The doctors conducting this research were greatly impressed with this result, and concluded that lowering blood-cholesterol levels by 25 per cent could cut heart-disease rates by half.

Not all experts would be quite so optimistic, but nearly all are convinced that lowering cholesterol is potentially a major life-saver. A recent worldwide survey of over 200 leading authorities on heart-disease prevention has found that 98 per cent accept the link between blood cholesterol and the development of coronary heart disease.

What's more, one of the most prestigious health organisations in the world, the United States National Institutes of Health, convened a panel of experts to study all the evidence concerning this crucial link. Their verdict, as far as those of us in the Western world are concerned, is that *for every 1 per cent reduction in blood cholesterol, there's a 2 per cent reduction in coronary heart-disease risk*.

The British Regional Heart Study

An important source of information on the causes of heart disease, at least in men, is a study of 7735 men aged 40–59, selected at random from general practitioners' lists in 24 towns throughout England, Wales and Scotland.

These men were subjected to a very thorough medical examination, including measurement of their height, weight, blood pressure, blood lipids and an ECG (electrocardiogram or heart-trace). They were also asked a string of questions about their eating, drinking, smoking, exercise and other habits. Five years later, they were asked the same questions, and their health has continued to be monitored ever since.

As with the Framingham Study, much valuable information on the risk factors for heart disease has been gleaned.

HDL: lowering the risk

We saw earlier that HDL – high-density lipoprotein – is the one and only fatty constituent of the blood which evidently has a beneficial effect on the health of the arteries. Laboratory studies have shown that this lipid is a form of cholesterol being carried away from the tissues, including the arterial walls, back to the liver for recycling. Measuring the HDL level gives an indication of how actively this protective process is going on. Higher levels have been found to be associated with a slower development of atheroma.

These findings have been borne out by large-scale studies on whole populations. The Framingham Study, for example, clearly demonstrated that people with higher levels of HDL do indeed have fewer heart attacks and angina than those with lower levels. Another example is the British Regional Heart Study, which has shown that middle-aged men with the highest HDLs have *half* the risk of those with the lowest. Similar results are emerging from other large studies around the world.

Unfortunately, the evidence suggests that the protective effect of a high HDL is not as powerful as the damaging effect of a high total cholesterol level. Nevertheless, anything which helps to boost your HDL at least helps to counteract the blood cholesterol effect.

The main factors which have so far been shown to raise HDL are a diet high in monounsaturated fats and regular aerobic-type exercise. The main factor lowering it is cigarette smoking.

Fibrinogen

There's increasing evidence that a protein in our blood may be as important an indicator of coronary and stroke risk as cholesterol.

Fibrinogen is a key substance in the clotting process, and vital in the prevention of haemorrhages. But a high level tends to make the blood more viscous (sticky) so that it doesn't flow so well through smaller arteries.

Studies have shown that people with higher levels of fibrinogen are more at risk of heart attacks and strokes. It's likely that because the blood is more viscous, it drags the delicate lining cells from the arterial walls, rather like a gale lifting roof slates. This initial damage is then followed by the beginnings of an atheroma plaque.

Having both high cholesterol and high fibrinogen is probably the worst combination of all, especially if the person is also a cigarette smoker or has high blood pressure.

A high fibrinogen also makes thrombosis more likely – again increasing the risk of a heart attack or stroke.

Factors which reduce blood stickiness – such as aspirin – or inhibit clotting, or encourage clot removal, are likely to have a beneficial effect in both of these conditions.

Cigarette smoking

There's no doubt that smoking cigarettes pushes up your risk of heart disease. A famous study of 34 440 male British doctors, followed up for 20 years, showed very clearly that their risk of a heart attack increased in direct parallel with the number of cigarettes they smoked a day. Smoking was found to be particularly dangerous for the hearts of younger men.

It's also been estimated that smoking causes about half the coronary deaths among middle-aged women.

In the Framingham Study, the heart-disease rate among smokers of either sex was two or three times that for people who had never smoked.

The British Regional Heart Study found a similar tripling of heart-disease risk for male smokers, and also confirmed that another crucial factor is how long the smoker has had the habit. The longer you've been a smoker, the higher your risk of heart disease.

International studies, such as the Seven Countries Study, suggest that the heart-threatening effect of smoking is worst in those populations with a relatively high average blood-cholesterol level – which is most Western nations.

In individuals, smoking combined with a high blood cholesterol and high blood pressure multiplies the heart-disease risk by up to eight times.

Many studies based on autopsies show that smoking markedly increases atherosclerosis, although why it does so is not clear. Smoking has relatively little effect on blood cholesterol and only slightly lowers HDL levels.

Smoking and thrombosis

Recent studies have shown that the main way in which smoking can influence your risk of having a heart attack is through its effect on blood viscosity (stickiness) and the tendency for blood to clot. The evidence suggests that smoking increases the level of fibrinogen in the blood. The higher the fibrinogen, the more viscous the blood – and the more likely it is to form a clot (thrombosis) in an already atheroma-damaged artery. This would account for the higher rate of heart attacks (coronary thrombosis) and strokes (cerebral thrombosis) amongst smokers.

This increase in stickiness and tendency to clot can be reversed within a week or two of giving up smoking. Some studies show a halving of the risk of a fatal heart attack within a year.

Smoking and heart disease

* Cigarette smoking is a major risk factor for heart disease, and has its most damaging effects in the younger age-groups.

* Smoking causes more premature deaths from heart disease than it does from lung diseases like cancer and emphysema.

* Men under 45 who smoke 25 cigarettes a day multiply their risk of a fatal heart attack by 15 times!

* Seven out of 10 coronary patients under 65 are smokers.

* Smokers who stop smoking can halve their risk of fatal coronary heart disease within a year.

Blood pressure

High blood pressure is a major risk factor for heart disease and strokes. The higher your blood pressure, the greater your risk.

The evidence for this comes from large-scale research studies following the health of thousands of people over many years.

For example, the Framingham Study involving 2-yearly

health checks on 5000 people for over 35 years, has found that people with high blood pressure have at least three times the risk of a heart attack compared with those with normal blood pressure. Even people whose blood pressure is on the borderline between normal and high have double the risk.

The British Regional Heart Study, following nearly 8000 men for more than 5 years, has also found that high blood pressure at least doubles the risk of a heart attack – and that men with the highest pressures have three times the risk.

What's more, several major studies, including these two, have shown that people with high blood pressure are running up to seven times the risk of having a stroke.

Various factors can push up our blood pressure: being overweight, eating too much sodium (mainly as salt) or drinking too much alcohol, for example. In Western countries like Britain, it also tends to rise as we get older.

For advice on how to keep your blood pressure under control, turn to page 109.

Multiple risk factors

The three main risk factors – high blood cholesterol, cigarette smoking and high blood pressure – work hand-in-hand to do mischief to the arteries, increasing the fatty deposits of atherosclerosis and hence the risk of heart attacks and strokes.

For someone who has any two, or all three, of these risk factors in combination, the risks aren't just added together – they're *multiplied*.

So, if you're a smoker with high blood pressure your risk is doubled and doubled again – in other words, it's quadrupled.

And if, on top of that, you're found to have a high blood

cholesterol, that's double the risk again. Your chances of a heart attack are *eight times more* than they would be without these risk factors.

Fortunately, you can do something about all three of these factors.

Lack of exercise

There's no shortage of evidence to support the advice that regular exercise is good for you. Literally hundreds of scientific papers attest to its health benefits.

Fitness helps to improve your suppleness, your strength and your staying power. It helps to keep you slim – or at least slimmer! It tones up your heart and circulation, preventing your heart rate and blood pressure from soaring whenever you get emotional, excited or exert yourself. It has beneficial effects on the lipids in your blood – reducing triglycerides and increasing HDL. And it helps to combat stress, making you feel good. (Yes, there's scientific evidence proving that you enjoy exercise!)

But what about the lack of exercise as a risk factor for heart disease?

This has been more difficult to investigate because, unlike the fitness benefits, which can all be achieved within a few weeks, the bonus in terms of avoiding heart attacks and strokes may take years to show itself.

Nevertheless, there are several long-term research studies which demonstrate, at least for men, a clear link between the amount of regular, moderately vigorous physical activity the subjects had, at work or leisure, and their subsequent risk of heart disease. The link isn't as powerful as it is for blood cholesterol, blood pressure or smoking – and can be easily overwhelmed by any of these – but it's definitely there none the less.

Studies of 3686 San Francisco dockworkers (1951–72)

and nearly 17 000 Harvard graduates (1962–72) have shown that men who have a moderate amount of regular, fairly vigorous exercise are less likely to succumb to heart attacks in later life. With the dockworkers, the exercise was moderate daily activity at work, burning up more than 8500 calories a week. With the graduates, it was leisure activity, burning up more than 2000 calories a week.

A study of more than 18 000 British male civil servants (1968–79) also looked at leisure activity, and found that the group who took vigorous exercise had far fewer coronaries later on – between one-third and one-half of the heart-attack rate suffered by the non-exercisers.

Unfortunately, similar studies for women, on such a large scale with such a long follow-up, have yet to be undertaken.

This is not because of a lack of interest in women's risks of heart disease. Rather, it's because women have far fewer heart attacks than men and it's much quicker (and therefore less expensive) to get statistically significant results by studying the latter.

Nevertheless, the shorter-term health benefits such as a lowered blood pressure and heart-rate response, an increase in HDL, lower triglycerides and improved weight control have been demonstrated in women who exercise regularly.

So, the clear message for both sexes is to keep moving. And there's advice on how to be more physical – sensibly, safely and enjoyably – in Chapter 7.

Weight

It's a well-established fact that overweight people are more at risk of heart disease and strokes.

For example, the Framingham Study showed that, among men aged 35–44, those whose weight was 10 per cent above the 'normal' for their height, had a 38 per cent higher risk of coronary heart disease – and those who were 20 per cent overweight had nearly double the risk.

The British Regional Heart Study of middle-aged men found a similar excess risk linked to excess body weight.

Statistical analysis of these and other research studies shows that the added heart-disease and stroke risk caused by being overweight is not so much a direct effect of all that flab. It is due more to the high blood pressure and high blood cholesterol that so often accompany a weight problem. Another risk factor for heart disease and strokes, namely diabetes, is also much commoner among overweight people – as is a lack of regular, vigorous exercise.

So being overweight is very likely to be bad news for your heart and arteries – usually for several different reasons – which makes it all the more important to keep as close as you can to your target weight range for your height (see page 89).

About alcohol

Much joy has greeted the finding that a little alcohol may have a beneficial effect on the heart. Several research studies suggest that a moderate intake over a period of years may be linked to a lower risk of coronary heart disease. In particular, moderate drinkers seem to suffer fewer coronaries than either heavy drinkers or, somewhat surprisingly, non-drinkers.

The fact that heavy drinking is bad for the heart is well known. But what can be bad about non-drinking?

On closer inspection it appears that people who don't drink, particularly men, usually have a reason for not doing so. It may be religious or cultural. But it may also be because they have an illness (perhaps a previous heart disease) which prevents them from enjoying alcohol, or because they have had a drink problem in the past. Moderate or light social drinkers also tend to be more health-conscious in all sorts of ways, and the key factor in their lower risk of heart disease may not be their level of drinking.

We do know that drinking, even just two drinks a day, can increase beneficial HDL levels in women – but not in men. On the other hand, moderate or heavy alcohol consumption can raise blood pressure, which increases the risk of heart disease and strokes.

Needless to say, alcohol is neat calories, and will definitely add to the problems of anyone who is overweight.

We've included advice on drinking 'well' in Chapter 7.

Stress

Most people firmly believe that stress is the main cause of heart attacks. Opinion polls put it way above an unhealthy diet, smoking or sloth as the heart's arch-enemy. But the backing for this belief has been very difficult to support scientifically.

One problem is that we all have different interpretations of the word 'stress'.

For some, it means tension or anxiety – with white knuckles, a dry mouth, a knotted throat and a pounding heart. For others, it's more like constant pressure, a heavy feeling of being weighed down by worries and unable to escape. And all of us feel stress at times of great difficulty or trauma: being made redundant, going through a divorce, losing a close friend or relative, buying a house – or even having three children under five.

The crucial aspect of stress, as far as your heart and arteries are concerned, is not so much the situation that causes it but how you react to it. What does stress do to your blood pressure, pulse rate, cholesterol level and the risk of thrombosis?

Experiments on human volunteers have shown that many people react to tension and anxiety by producing more so-called 'fight or flight' hormones – adrenalin and noradrenalin – whose main effects on the blood and circulation are to increase blood pressure and pulse rate, raise the total cholesterol level, lower the 'beneficial' HDL level and increase the stickiness of blood, making it more prone to clotting.

But demonstrating a link between these short-term physiological changes and long-term atherosclerosis, heart disease and strokes has not been easy. One of the main difficulties has been in deriving a standard measure of stress or an individual's reaction to it (as described in Chapter 4).

Nevertheless, there is almost certainly a link between stressful events and the risk of a heart attack in people whose coronary arteries are already narrowed with atheroma. The great eighteenth-century anatomist, John Hunter, who suffered from angina, once said that his life was in the hands of any rascal who vexed him. During a violent argument at Guy's Hospital he clutched his chest and died on the spot.

Diabetes

The Framingham Study has found that people with diabetes have double the risk of dying from heart disease, although whether this is due to the diabetes or its link with high blood cholesterol is not clear. In countries whose people have a low rate of coronary heart disease, and low blood-cholesterol levels, the presence of diabetes does not seem to add to the risk.

Nevertheless, in the Western world, where cholesterol levels are generally high, diabetes is definitely an additional hazard. People who have this condition should make every effort to keep their risk factors as low as possible, especially their cholesterol level.

Gout

People with gout tend to have an increased risk of heart disease. The evidence suggests that there is a link between having a high level of uric acid in the blood (the basic metabolic disorder underlying the symptoms of gout) and having a high blood-cholesterol level.

The reason for this is not fully understood.

Family history

It's a well-established fact that heart disease and strokes have an unfortunate tendency to run in families – at least to some extent. For example, a heart attack under the age of 50 in a close blood relative (parent, child or sibling) can multiply your own risk by up to four times.

This genetic susceptibility – the 'family effect' – is usually very complex, involving a great many genes and several major risk factors. Obesity, high blood pressure and diabetes can, in some families, be passed down from generation to generation. Certainly, the tendency to have a high blood cholesterol is something that can run quite strongly in families. All in all, it has been estimated that perhaps about one-third of the average person's risk of premature heart disease or stroke is due to inherited factors, and two-thirds to other factors, of which far and away the most important is their diet.

But the blood-cholesterol level in an unfortunate tiny minority is overwhelmingly affected by a single abnormal gene. This is the basis of the inherited disorder called 'familial hypercholesterolaemia' (see page 56).

— 4 —

What Makes Your Cholesterol Rise . . . or Fall?

There's a long list of factors that can play a part in determining your level of cholesterol.

Some of them are unavoidable like your age, sex and family history. For women, your cholesterol will depend on whether you're pregnant, or past your menopause.

Your body weight and level of aerobic fitness are important factors. Various medical conditions – like diabetes, an under-active thyroid gland and familial hypercholesterolaemia – can push your cholesterol level up. So, too, can a number of medications – like the contraceptive pill, certain drugs for high blood pressure and some types of steroid drugs.

But for most people, far and away the most crucial day-to-day influence on their cholesterol, and the one that they can most easily change for the better, is their diet – the effect of their everyday food and drink.

We shall look at this in detail a little later on. But first, let's consider some of the other factors more closely.

How do age and sex affect cholesterol?
In developed nations, the average person's cholesterol rises steadily as he or she gets older. This is usually not the case among people in developing countries – their cholesterol levels stay more or less constant throughout life. The reason for this difference is unknown, but is likely to be a

combination of genetic and environmental factors.

Your sex certainly influences your cholesterol – although the difference between men and women isn't huge, and it reverses in later life. Women have a slightly lower level under the age of 50, and a slightly higher level above that age. This sex difference is almost certainly linked to the level of female hormones before and after the menopause; but this is not enough, in itself, to explain the difference in risk of a heart attack between men and women.

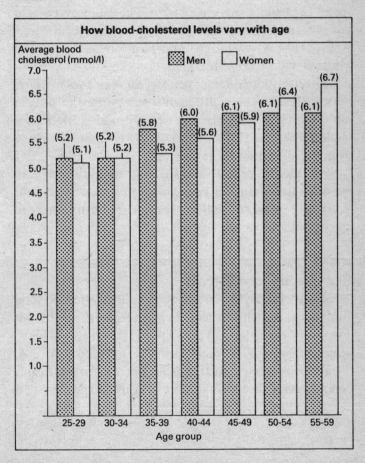

How blood-cholesterol levels vary with age

Average blood cholesterol (mmol/l) — Men, Women

Age group: 25-29, 30-34, 35-39, 40-44, 45-49, 50-54, 55-59

Men: (5.2), (5.2), (5.8), (6.0), (6.1), (6.1), (6.1)
Women: (5.1), (5.2), (5.3), (5.6), (5.9), (6.4), (6.7)

And pregnancy?

Hormones again play a crucial part here. As pregnancy hormones increase they temporarily raise blood cholesterol and triglycerides to ensure adequate supplies to the developing foetus.

The levels usually subside again within a few weeks of the birth.

Obesity and cholesterol

Another possible factor is obesity. The more overweight you are, the higher your blood cholesterol is likely to be. Being very overweight can also push down the level of HDL, the 'protective' blood lipid.

Conversely, the slimmer you are, the lower your cholesterol is likely to be – although it's important to bear in mind the many other factors which can also affect your cholesterol level. Thin people are by no means immune from having a high cholesterol.

Nevertheless, because keeping your weight under control is so important for your health in general, and your heart in particular, we'll be considering it in depth in Chapter 7.

Exercise and cholesterol

Although exercise has no appreciable direct effect on total cholesterol, it helps to reduce triglycerides in the blood, and increases the level of protective HDL. It also helps to keep your weight and blood pressure under control.

Needless to say, regular exercise has many other health benefits, which we look at more fully in Chapter 7.

Stress and cholesterol

We all have our own ideas about stress: what it means, and how it can affect us. Many people think of it as a form of chronic anxiety or pressure, a continuous burden or strain, that takes its toll of our health in several different ways ranging from skin rashes and bowel upsets to high blood pressure and heart disease. Others see stress as a sudden shock or loss, which 'pulls the rug from under you' and leads to a nervous depression and inability to cope. Still others see stress more in terms of how a particular individual is reacting in general to life's demands. Are they on top of things, or are they going under? One person's stress is another person's stimulation.

Measuring stress

Medically speaking, there's no clear definition as to precisely what 'stress' is. This, of course, makes it very difficult to measure, and hence doubly difficult to research. How can we investigate the effects of stress on, say, blood-cholesterol levels without knowing exactly how much stress is involved?

There have been some attempts to quantify it. The main type of measure that's been developed is a standard questionnaire which asks people a long list of questions about their personality, their likes and dislikes, how they think they'd react in different circumstances, their psychological and physical health and so on. Their answers are then added up to give a score. A number of different questionnaires are available, each giving different scores on different aspects of an individual's personality or psychology. But as long as the same questionnaire is used in any particular comparison, the results will be reasonably valid.

Type A troubles

Using this approach, the possible link between stress – scientists prefer to say 'psycho-social factors' – and blood cholesterol has been investigated. In general, studies have shown that subjects whose personality falls into the so-called 'Type A' category – thrusting, aggressive, deadline-dominated, tense, jaw-grinding (you know the sort!) – tend to have higher levels of cholesterol and lower levels of protective HDL. Perhaps more importantly, their blood is stickier and more likely to clot, predisposing to thrombosis. They also tend to have higher blood pressure and are more likely to be smokers. All of these are risk factors for heart disease, and some are risk factors for strokes.

Being able to cope with stressful situations is clearly important for health, and you can find practical guidelines in Chapter 7.

Diabetes and cholesterol

Men and women with diabetes tend to have a higher level of blood cholesterol than other people and find it harder to keep their cholesterol down. They also tend to have a lower level of protective HDL. However, these effects only partly explain why people with diabetes have a much higher risk of heart disease than the rest of the population. The full story is still unknown.

Nevertheless, keeping the blood-glucose level under control helps to lower the cholesterol level and reduce that risk.

An under-active thyroid gland

An under-active thyroid gland – also known as myxoedema or hypothyroidism – can push the level of cholesterol sky-high. The condition most commonly affects middle-aged women, causing hair loss, coarse facial features, gruff voice, mental and physical slowness and an increase in weight. These effects are due to the lack of thyroid hormone (thyroxine), which also causes the cholesterol increase. Treatment with thyroxine usually brings about a dramatic improvement of the symptoms, and a marked reduction in cholesterol.

Gout and cholesterol

People with gout – a form of arthritis caused by a raised uric-acid level in the blood – usually also have a high blood cholesterol. Successful prevention or treatment of the gout with uric-acid-lowering drugs usually also lowers their cholesterol.

Can some medication increase cholesterol?

Indeed, yes. Many therapeutic drug treatments may do just that. Here are some commonly prescribed examples.

The most widely used is the Pill – the combined oral contraceptive. This is a combination of synthetic oestrogen and a synthetic progesterone-type hormone (progestogen) – the two hormones involved in the menstrual cycle. The relatively high doses that were used in older brands of the Pill tended to cause an increase in blood pressure, susceptibility to thrombosis and a slight increase in blood cholesterol in some women – especially those over the age of 35, and even more especially those who smoked. However, modern formulations of the Pill contain much lower doses of hormones, and are much less likely to lead to these changes. Most recent studies suggest that cholesterol is hardly affected, and that some versions of the Pill may actually increase protective HDL in the blood. The so-called 'minipill' contraceptive – the progestogen-only

Pill – also seems to have a beneficial effect on HDL.

Thiazide diuretics – urine-stimulating medication used widely for controlling high blood pressure – can increase cholesterol levels. This is important because many people with high blood pressure also have a high blood cholesterol – often without themselves or their doctor knowing about it. If they are given a thiazide diuretic, their blood cholesterol is likely to rise even higher.

Another type of medication used for high blood pressure, so-called 'beta blockers', can also cause a raised blood cholesterol. However, the newer, more specifically cardiac-acting beta blockers don't seem to have this effect.

Corticosteroids, whose anti-inflammatory effect is used to treat certain forms of arthritis and other chronic inflammatory diseases, can lead to a raised blood cholesterol – as can a certain type of anti-acne medication, tretinoin.

Familial hypercholesterolaemia

This disorder – otherwise known as FH or Family Heart Disease – is one of a group of inherited disorders affecting the balance of lipids (fatty substances) in the blood. It is estimated that, in most Western societies, up to one person in 300 has one of these disorders, and about one person in 500 has FH in particular.

Basic fault

The basic fault, caused by a single defective gene, lies in the special proteins in the plasma that transport lipids such as cholesterol and triglycerides from place to place in the body. These proteins, called 'apoproteins', combine with lipids to form lipoproteins (see Chapter 2). FH causes an imbalance of apoproteins, which in turn alters the levels of cholesterol, HDL and triglycerides in the blood.

Sky-high cholesterol

From childhood onwards, people with FH have an extremely high blood cholesterol – in some cases, about three times the normal level! – although, because there are no immediate symptoms, they're usually completely unaware of the time-bomb lurking in their arteries.

Young victims

As you might imagine, FH carries a dramatically increased risk of coronary heart disease and, to some extent, strokes. It can multiply the odds of having a heart attack by eight or more times. What's especially tragic is that it speeds up and intensifies the whole process of atherosclerosis (furring up of the arteries), so that constrictions and blockages occur much earlier in life than normal. People with untreated FH usually succumb to severe angina and heart attacks in early middle age, instead of the more usual late middle age or old age. Indeed, when men have the disorder disaster often strikes in their 30s or even 20s.

Cholesterol clues

Apart from having a very high blood cholesterol, and close relatives who have suffered from heart disease at an early age, the only other clues someone with FH is likely to provide is in the form of cholesterol deposits at various places around the body. For instance, yellowish lumps may appear in the tendons – particularly the Achilles tendons above the heels, and the tendons on the backs of the hands and wrists. Similar yellowish lumps may arise under the skin of the elbows, in the creases of the palms of the hands and, most commonly, in the thin skin of the eyelids or corner of the eye. Cholesterol may also be deposited in the eye itself – in a whitish ring around the edge of the cornea, the normally clear round window over the coloured iris and pupil.

However, although they are important clues, these deposits of cholesterol don't necessarily mean that the person has FH or a similar inherited disorder. In fact, the deposits in and around the eye are quite common in middle-aged or older people without FH, whose blood cholesterol is only moderately high. But if they occur in someone under the age of 50, they're a useful clue to FH – and if the person is under 30, they're a pretty sure sign.

Urgent action

Anyone with a 'bad' family history of heart disease (especially if a parent, brother or sister suffered angina, heart attack or sudden death under the age of 55) should have their cholesterol measured. If it's very high, and they themselves have children, the children should also have the test.

The first approach to treatment is a cholesterol-lowering, low-fat, fibre-rich diet (as outlined in Chapter 8). If this doesn't bring the cholesterol down enough, drug treatment may be necessary (see page 118). Really severe cases may need repeated courses of a special blood-filtering treatment, apheresis, every fortnight. This removes large amounts of cholesterol whilst leaving the protective HDL undisturbed.

— 5 —

Food and Your Cholesterol

For the great majority of us, by far the most important factor affecting our blood cholesterol on a day-to-day, week-by-week basis is what we eat – especially the balance of the different types of fat in our food and drink.

There are literally thousands of scientific papers on the subject of diet and its effects on blood cholesterol, other blood lipids, heart disease and strokes. Clearly, these can't be summarised in a few short paragraphs. This section looks at the main evidence, and those conclusions which are most important as far as healthy eating is concerned.

'Mr Fit'

This huge research study in the United States of America, properly called the Multiple Risk Factor Intervention Trial (MRFIT), but better known as the 'Mr Fit Study', involved 12 866 men aged 35–57, who were selected as being at high risk of succumbing to heart disease.

The men were divided into two groups. One received firm instructions to eat a healthy diet and stop smoking, with check-ups every 4 months – whilst members of the other were given their usual annual medical without any special advice.

Although the men in both groups took steps to improve their health, after 7 years the group given the special programme had a lower average blood cholesterol, lower blood pressure, smoked less – and had fewer heart attacks.

The fat factor

In Chapter 2, we saw how most of the cholesterol in our blood is synthesised in the liver from the breakdown products of fats and oils in our diet. Usually, only a minor proportion comes directly from *cholesterol* in our food.

Apart from dietary cholesterol, nearly all the dozens of different fats and oils in our food are members of the same chemical family: triglycerides. The only real difference between fats and oils is that oils are liquid at room temperature, whereas fats are solid or semi-solid.

All triglycerides are built of fatty acids combined with glycerol. There are many different fatty acids, but they each belong to one of three 'families' depending on their chemical structure: saturated, monounsaturated or poly-unsaturated. The precise meanings of these terms needn't concern us here, but the proportions of each type in the different fats and oils we eat make a big difference to the way these foods are handled by the body – particularly the effect they have on blood-cholesterol levels.

Saturated fats

Fats or oils that are high in saturated fatty acids, sometimes referred to as 'saturated fats', are found mainly in foods of animal origin – meat and meat products, milk, butter and other dairy produce – but also in some plant oils, most notably palm oil, coconut oil and 'hardened' (hydrogenated) vegetable oils. Saturated fats are solid or semi-solid at room temperature.

It's now firmly established, through experiments with animals and humans, and by observing whole populations, that a diet high in saturated fats tends to increase blood-cholesterol levels, and hence the risk of a heart attack or stroke. There's also ample evidence that cutting down on saturated fats reduces your blood cholesterol.

> ### *Milk and butter 'flutter'*
>
> There has been controversy in Britain recently as to whether the advice to reduce full-fat milk and butter consumption, as a rich source of saturated fats, is scientifically justifiable. A research study on nearly 5000 men aged 45–59, followed for several years, seemed to indicate that men drinking more full-fat milk and eating more butter had *lower* rates of heart disease than men who avoided these foods – apparently turning the usual advice completely on its head!
>
> However, on closer examination it was found that the men who avoided high-fat milk and butter were likely to be more worried about having a heart attack because they had heart disease in their family or because they'd experienced heart-disease symptoms themselves. Not surprisingly, these men were bound to be most at risk, whatever they ate or drank.

Monounsaturated fats

Many fats and oils of both plant and animal origin are high in monounsaturates. These include olive, peanut and rape-seed oil. Most monounsaturated fats are liquid at room temperature, but become semi-solid in the refrigerator.

The balance of scientific evidence so far suggests that monounsaturates are fairly neutral with regard to their effect on total blood cholesterol. Nevertheless, if a highly monounsaturated fat, such as olive oil, is used to replace a highly saturated fat, such as palm oil or lard, this will certainly help to reduce the blood cholesterol.

What's more, there's now good evidence to show that monounsaturates do have a direct benefit in their own right – they help to boost protective HDL and hence have an anti-atheroma effect. This could explain why some Mediterranean countries like southern Italy and Greece, whose cooking uses plenty of olive oil, have such a low incidence of heart disease.

Polyunsaturated fats

Fats and oils high in polyunsaturates include safflower oil, sunflower oil, soya oil, corn oil and most fish oils. Most polyunsaturated fats are liquid at room temperature, and remain liquid in the refrigerator.

Three polyunsaturates are essential for healthy nutrition – linoleic acid, linolenic acid and arachidonic acid. The first two are plentiful in various plant-seed oils, the last in small amounts in animal fats. Both linolenic and

---

Fish for health

What do Greenland Eskimos (Inuits) and the Japanese have in common? They both eat lots of fish and have very low heart-disease rates. What's more, the lowest rates in Japan are among the people of Okinawa, whose fish consumption is about twice that of mainland Japanese.

A study in the Netherlands measured people's fish consumption in 1960, and followed their health for 20 years. The researchers found a clear relationship between the amount of fish eaten and the risk of coronary heart disease: the higher the consumption, the lower the risk. In fact, mortality from heart attacks among those who ate at least 30 g (about 1 oz) of fish a day was less than half the rate among those who ate no fish at all.

Attention has focused on oily fish: sardines, tuna, mackerel, herring and salmon. These are high in polyunsaturated fats – and, in particular, the so-called 'long-chain omega-3' polyunsaturated fatty acids: eicosapentaenoic acid and docosahexaenoic acid (EPA and DHA for short).

These omega-3 fatty acids have been shown in the laboratory to inhibit blood-clot formation – an effect also found with some polyunsaturated fatty acids from plant seeds.

It's this clot-resistance, and hence the prevention of coronary and cerebral thrombosis, which could account for the life-saving potential of a diet high in polyunsaturates in general – and fish oils in particular.

---

arachidonic acids can be made by the body from linoleic acid, but it is truly essential to include this last fatty acid in our food – it can only be obtained from the diet. Fortunately, seed oils, particularly sunflower, contain lots of it.

Some research studies show that people with low levels of linoleic acid have a higher risk of heart disease. A recent study in Scotland, for example, found that men with the lowest levels of linoleic acid in their body fat had three times the risk of angina or a heart attack.

Quite why, or how, linoleic acid can reduce heart-disease risk is not yet known, but it may be linked to a lessening of early damage to the walls of arteries or a reduction in the stickiness of blood, minimising thrombosis.

Apart from these specific effects, polyunsaturates, like monounsaturates, also have the important function of providing a useful replacement for saturated fats in the diet – for instance, using plant oils high in polyunsaturates instead of lard for cooking, or using sunflower spread instead of butter.

For practical advice on how to reduce saturated fats in your food, and partly substitute unsaturated fats – mono or poly – turn to Chapter 8.

National differences

The Seven Countries Study showed very strikingly that populations with a high average level of blood cholesterol, in countries like Finland, the Netherlands and the United States, also have a diet high in saturated fats. These are mainly of animal origin, such as the fat in meat and meat products, and in milk and dairy products. What's more, these high-saturated-fat countries also had high rates of coronary heart disease.

By contrast, the countries such as Japan, Italy and Greece, with lower saturated-fat intakes – whose inhabitants instead ate a higher proportion of monounsaturated or polyunsaturated fats (mainly of plant, fish or poultry origin) – had lower blood cholesterols and lower heart-disease incidence rates.

Other comparisons between different populations have found the same link: the more saturated fat in the diet, and the lower the proportion of unsaturated fats, the higher the risk of coronary heart disease.

Comparing individuals

A number of large-scale studies have shown that this link holds true for individuals. Broadly speaking, people who eat a lot of saturated fat, and insufficient monounsaturated or polyunsaturated fat, are more at risk of heart disease.

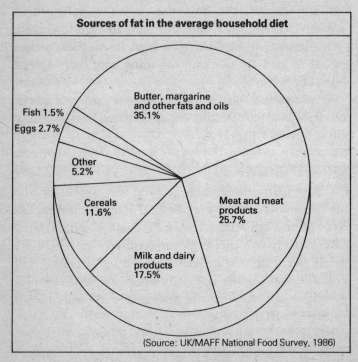

Sources of fat in the average household diet

Butter, margarine and other fats and oils 35.1%

Fish 1.5%

Eggs 2.7%

Other 5.2%

Cereals 11.6%

Meat and meat products 25.7%

Milk and dairy products 17.5%

(Source: UK/MAFF National Food Survey, 1986)

For example, a study followed the health of nearly 2000 employees of Western Electric in Chicago for 20 years, and found that those who developed angina or had heart attacks tended to have high-saturated-fat diets. A very similar finding emerged in Britain from an 11-year study of nearly 20 000 male civil servants.

The message about fat

All in all, most of the evidence points to one conclusion: too much saturated fat, and too little monounsaturated or polyunsaturated fat, is likely to put up your risk of atherosclerosis, heart disease or a stroke.

Everybody's different

Nevertheless, as far as the individual person is concerned, although their heart-disease risk may be increased – perhaps greatly increased – this doesn't mean that they will definitely have trouble. We still have no certain way of predicting what will happen to any particular person. Everybody's different, and there are undoubtedly some people who eat a diet high in saturated fat for decades without ever getting a high cholesterol level. Equally, there are some people whose cholesterol is through the roof, and yet they escape angina, a heart attack or a stroke.

These exceptions to the rule at least serve to remind us that even allowing for other known risk factors, such as smoking habits, blood pressure or exercise levels, there are certain individual mechanisms that determine how your body will react to the fats in your food. Your genes certainly make a difference – and scientists are getting close to being able to pinpoint, using genetic material, those people who have heart disease 'programmed' into their future health.

Coffee

There's been some concern recently that coffee-drinking may increase the risk of heart disease. In a number of studies, heart-attack victims have been asked lots of questions about their lifestyle, and their answers compared with those of other people who haven't had a heart attack. Among the many differences, it looks at first sight as though there's a link between coffee-drinking and having a heart attack.

But a closer look at the data has shown that this link is not very clear-cut. Nor is there good evidence that it's causal – at the moment, it's merely a statistical association.

Nevertheless, strong black coffee made from boiled ground beans does seem to be linked with a high total cholesterol level in the blood – five or six cups a day can have a marked effect. By contrast, instant coffee has a very small cholesterol-raising effect. The same is true of decaffeinated coffee or tea.

So, if you've got a high cholesterol, it's probably sensible to cut right down on strong coffee and switch to a milder, more artery-friendly beverage.

Cholesterol in food

So far we've concentrated on the role of fats in your food, and how they may affect your blood-cholesterol level and other key factors with regard to heart disease and stroke.

But what about dietary cholesterol – the cholesterol that's actually present in the food you eat? Surely, eating dietary cholesterol is bound to push up the level in the blood, isn't it? Too much dietary cholesterol can't be good for you.

As we saw in Chapter 2, about 90 per cent of the body's cholesterol is made internally from building blocks derived from the fat you eat. Only 10 per cent comes directly from cholesterol in your food. This means that the most important dietary changes you need to make concern the fat content in your diet – eat less fat altogether, and replace foods high in saturates with others high in monounsaturates and polyunsaturates.

It's certainly worth reducing dietary cholesterol as well – but because most of it is in the same sorts of foods as saturated fat, namely meat and dairy products, this will happen anyway when you change your diet.

True, some foods are especially high in dietary cholesterol. Examples are egg yolks, liver, kidney, brain, prawns and some other shellfish. But, apart from eggs, you're unlikely to be eating large quantities of these foods in comparison with the total amount of fat you eat. It is rather too easy to eat too many egg yolks – in cake mixes, batters and salad dressings as well as in whole eggs – so it is worth keeping a check on them. No more than four a week, which includes eggs used in cake mixes, etc.

Fibre

Much interest has recently surrounded the possible role of dietary fibre in lowering blood-cholesterol levels.

We've all become familiar with fibre over the past few years, as nutritionists have come to understand how important it is in a healthy diet. It's essentially the largely indigestible parts of the food we obtain from plants – cell walls (mainly cellulose), gums, gels and pectins – in cereals (especially wholegrain), vegetables, fruit and nuts.

Fibre has long been known to improve digestion and help prevent constipation. 'Eat plenty of roughage to keep your bowels moving' has been the byword in the developed world for at least a century or two – and there's abundant evidence that a fibre-rich diet does indeed speed up the movement of waste through the large intestine, and add bulk and softness to the stools.

But over the past 20 years, interest has focused on the

> **Get your oats!**
> Good sources of soluble fibre include beans, peas, lentils, chick peas, broccoli, spinach, cabbage, berries and other fruit and vegetables. Another excellent source is oats. Most of the soluble fibre in oats is in the bran – so one way of bumping up your soluble-fibre intake is to add oatbran (obtainable from wholefood and health food shops and some supermarkets) to porridge, muesli and baking mixes. Several brands of breakfast cereal are also now available with added oatbran.

potential role of a fibre-rich diet in preventing a whole range of other disorders, from dental decay to varicose veins, including atherosclerosis and heart disease.

There are two main types of fibre, soluble and insoluble.

Soluble fibre

Soluble fibre consists of plant substances which dissolve in the watery contents of the alimentary tract, but are not digested and broken down enough to be absorbed into the bloodstream. Instead, they form a sticky, jelly-like solution which is then worked on by the normal bacterial population in the bowel, and passed out of the body.

These substances are mainly gums, gels and pectins and are most abundant in the flesh of fruit, leafy vegetables, pulses (like beans, peas, lentils, chick peas) and some cereals, notably oats (particularly in oatbran).

These substances aren't obviously fibrous – but, as far as your cholesterol is concerned, they are the most important kind of fibre.

Insoluble fibre

This type of fibre is more obvious 'roughage'. It consists of tough substances which comprise the cell-walls of plants, and which don't dissolve at all in the alimentary tract. Instead of being digested they swell with water and add bulk to the stools, helping to prevent constipation and bowel disorders such as diverticulitis and bowel cancer.

The main substances in insoluble fibre are chewy cellulose, bulky hemicellulose and woody lignin. They are found mostly in wholegrain cereals (particularly in the bran) but also to some extent in pulses and vegetables.

Fibre and cholesterol

As you'll remember from Chapter 2, most of the cholesterol in our bodies is synthesised in the liver from fat in our diet, and most of that cholesterol is used to make bile, the digestive system's fat-dissolving 'washing-up liquid'. Bile is stored in the gall bladder and squirted into the duodenum (the first part of the intestine) after a fatty meal. When it has done its job, most of it is re-absorbed in the large intestine and returned to the liver for recycling, reducing the amount of cholesterol that has to be re-synthesised.

The theory goes that if we can somehow prevent the bile constituents (mainly acidic salts) from being re-absorbed, they will pass out of the body and be lost. The liver will therefore be forced to use up more cholesterol to make the necessary bile, and the blood-cholesterol level will fall.

With this idea in mind, scientists started to look very hard at food substances which might retain bile salts and prevent them being re-absorbed. They soon discovered that fibre, but especially soluble fibre, has this important property – it forms a sticky, jelly-like solution which mops up the bile salts and retains them, in the same way that a party jelly holds its colour. The fibre, together with the bile salts, then passes out of the body in the stools.

Experiments involving people eating diets rich in soluble fibre have confirmed that their blood-cholesterol level does indeed fall, by 10–25 per cent, after a few weeks. This would help to explain why people who eat lots of fruit, vegetables and pulses (such as southern Italians and Greeks, as well as vegetarians) have lower cholesterol levels and less heart disease.

Garlic charm?

The medicinal folklore surrounding garlic is legendary, and there can be few disorders that haven't apparently been miraculously cured or alleviated by this pungent herb. In the past few years, scientific evidence has been mounting to support some of the more consistent claims made for it.

In particular, there's now fairly convincing evidence that garlic can reduce cholesterol levels. Several recent studies have shown that over a period of a few months garlic, either fresh or as oil, or in tablets of the powdered concentrate, can bring down total cholesterol by 11–18 per cent. Triglycerides (fats in blood) are also reduced – and there's an increase in the level of 'beneficial' HDL. Other studies suggest that garlic may also have clot-dissolving properties.

Could all these effects help to explain why some Mediterranean countries, such as southern France, Italy and Greece, have such low rates of coronary heart disease?

Probably not, because quite large daily doses are needed to bring about these changes – equivalent to 30 g (just over 1 oz) of raw garlic clove every day. Not surprisingly, many people taking this amount, even in the form of tablets, have a strong whiff of garlic on their breath. So far, deodorised tablets have not been shown to be as effective in reducing cholesterol and the substance that brings about the beneficial changes has not yet been clearly identified.

More research is needed on this. But, in the meantime,

The African experience

Most of the world's poorer communities eat a diet based mainly on cereals and vegetables. In parts of rural Africa, for example, the people depend mainly on cassava and maize for their staple food. About 30 years ago, a British naval doctor, Surgeon-Captain T. L. Cleave, working in East Africa, observed that the rural communities were much more likely than their city-dwelling cousins to be spared a number of diseases – notably coronary heart disease, high blood pressure, strokes, diabetes, gallstones, bowel disease, varicose veins and tooth decay.

Surgeon-Captain Cleave came to the conclusion that these differences could be explained by the different diets of rural and urban Africans. Rural Africans eat less meat, less sugar and many more unrefined foods of plant origin than the city-dwellers. He was particularly impressed by the huge difference in the amount of unrefined carbohydrate food – high-fibre starchy cereals, vegetables, fruit and nuts – eaten by the two communities, and was convinced that this could account for all the differences in their susceptibility to that long list of 'diseases of affluence'.

Dietary studies elsewhere in the world have confirmed this view. People on a diet high in fibre-rich starchy foods do indeed tend to have less heart disease and strokes than those who eat little fibre – even after taking into account all sorts of other differences like smoking habits, stress levels and genetic differences.

you can happily prepare delicious meals with plenty of garlic, reasonably secure in the knowledge that it's at least helping to keep your cholesterol down.

Lecithin

This is the collective name for a group of fatty substances, all a form of phospholipid, present in the cells of all animals and plants. One of its main functions is to act as a 'wetting agent' or emulsifier. In egg yolks, for example, it helps to prevent the microscopic globules of fat from clumping together and separating out (or 'curdling'). It has a similar function in the human bloodstream.

Lecithin, derived chiefly from soya oil, is widely used in food manufacture as an emulsifier, particularly in low-fat

Vegetarians and cholesterol

Vegetarians are the obvious people to study in order to see the effect of fibre and other factors in a diet based mainly on cereals, pulses, vegetables and fruit.

A few large-scale studies comparing their health with that of non-vegetarians have been carried out – particularly in Britain and the United States. The American study followed the progress of 27 000 Seventh-day Adventists for 20 years to see whether their dietary habits had any connection with their subsequent health. Seventh-day Adventists advocate vegetarianism, although they don't insist on it. They do, however, insist on abstaining from smoking and drinking alcohol. The researchers found that Adventists who were vegetarian were much less likely to have heart disease than those who weren't – and that this applied to both sexes.

Careful studies elsewhere have shown that a vegetarian diet reduces blood cholesterol and blood pressure, both important risk factors for heart disease – although it's not yet clear whether this is due mainly to the exclusion of meat (thus cutting down on saturated fat) or eating great quantities of cereals, pulses, vegetables and fruit (containing lots of soluble fibre and the anti-oxidant Vitamins C and E).

Evidence from countries such as Greece and southern Italy, where meat is eaten together with plenty of bread, rice or pasta, and large amounts of vegetables and fresh fruit, suggests that both aspects play an important part, and that it's possible to derive the benefits of all those plant foods without necessarily giving up meat.

spreads and chocolate, and has its own E-number – E322. It can also be bought in health food shops.

There has been considerable interest in using lecithin to lower cholesterol. The theory was that the cholesterol would be suspended in the blood by the lecithin, and would therefore be less likely to be deposited in atheroma plaques.

This has not been borne out by research. One major problem is that when lecithin is eaten it's digested into simpler substances, which are then absorbed into the bloodstream and broken down in the liver. What's more, the body makes as much or as little lecithin as it needs.

So, back to the drawing board!

— 6 —
How High Is Your Cholesterol?

This chapter looks at how you can find out what your blood-cholesterol level is, and how you can work out what it means, together with other risk factors, in terms of your overall risk of heart disease.

How is blood cholesterol measured?

There are two main ways. One uses a drop of blood from a fingerprick and gives a result within a few minutes, but is not very accurate (desktop analysis). The other needs a syringe of blood from a vein, takes a day or two to get a result, but is much more accurate (laboratory lipid analysis).

Fingerprick test

This test has become widely available thanks to the development of a relatively inexpensive desktop machine which uses 'dry chemistry' and gives a digital reading.

The tip of your finger is pricked, and a small drop of blood is squeezed on to a specially impregnated strip which is then slotted into the analyser – a machine about the size and shape of a typewriter. After about 3 minutes of analysis, the machine provides a digital read-out of the total cholesterol level.

Rough and ready

Marvels of modern science and technology though they undoubtedly are, these desktop machines are not very sophisticated lipid analysers. At present, most of them can only measure total blood cholesterol – not HDL – and can't do the sort of full lipid analysis that you get from a laboratory test. They are highly delicate machines that have to be very carefully and frequently calibrated (zeroed) in order to give a reasonably accurate result. What's more, because they use blood from a fingertip capillary rather than a main vein, all sorts of factors may affect the validity of the reading.

Nevertheless, the fingerprick test, if done using a well-calibrated, well-maintained machine, can give you at least a rough idea of your cholesterol level – and, if proper advice is available, can be useful in motivating you to do something about your diet or smoking.

But if your reading is high you should ask your doctor to send a sample of your blood for a proper laboratory test.

Machines galore

Desktop machines are being actively marketed by their manufacturers, and many are being lent to doctors by pharmaceutical companies who make lipid-lowering drugs. Chemists' shops, health food shops, fitness centres and even some supermarkets now have cholesterol analysers. Medical experts are concerned that many of the machines deployed in these non-medical settings may not be properly calibrated or maintained, and that qualified advisers may not be on hand to interpret the results and give accurate, practical advice on the full range of heart-risk factors, including diet, exercise and smoking.

Laboratory lipid analysis

There are two versions of this test, both requiring a small syringeful of blood to be taken from a vein in your arm.

The first is a 'casual' or 'non-fasting' total cholesterol check. The sample is taken at any time of the day, and you don't have to starve yourself beforehand.

This is not a full lipid analysis but because it uses a larger quantity of blood from a main vein, and is analysed in properly standardised laboratory conditions, it gives a more accurate total measure of your total blood-cholesterol level than the fingerprick test.

The second version is a 'fasting' lipid profile. For this, you'll be asked to refrain from eating or drinking anything (apart from water or fruit juice) for about 12 hours before the sample is taken. Usually, you'll be asked to miss your late-night snack, bedtime drink and breakfast (including your morning cup of tea or coffee) before the test. This is to prevent the effect of fat in your food interfering with the blood-lipid results, particularly the triglyceride level, and making them difficult to interpret. By fasting, your lipid levels become much more standardised and comparable with results from other people and national averages.

A full blood-lipid profile gives not only your level of total cholesterol, but also your HDL and triglycerides, and perhaps your LDL as a separate measure. In other words, it provides a much more comprehensive picture of those circulating blood lipids which, together with other factors, can play such a crucial part in determining your risk of having a heart attack, angina or stroke.

However, a full lipid profile is not cheap, either to the National Health Service or to yourself if done privately, and is not necessary for most people with a moderately raised blood cholesterol. Your total blood-cholesterol level is only slightly affected by recent meals, and a casual test is usually quite adequate for most people.

Knowing your number

Since 1985, throughout the United States, every adult, healthy or otherwise, has been urged to have their cholesterol checked as part of a massive campaign run by the United States National Cholesterol Education Program. 'Know Your Number' is the slogan – the 'number' being your blood-cholesterol level – and the purpose has been to make people aware of the importance of cholesterol, together with other factors, in determining their risk of heart disease, and to provide dietary advice or treatment.

Mass screening

As you can imagine, this kind of 'mass screening' approach is very ambitious and very expensive to mount. It involves thousands of desktop analysers, with properly trained operators and lifestyle advisers, being set up in doctors' offices (surgeries), clinics, workplaces, shopping malls and leisure centres; special caravans or trailers are taken to shows, fairs, parades or any place where lots of people will be congregating. It's a huge undertaking – and latest estimates suggest that about two-thirds of adults in America have had their cholesterol checked.

Opportunistic screening

Another approach, which is far less costly to run, is so-called 'opportunistic screening'. This simply means that people are offered a test if and when they attend a surgery or clinic for any reason, whether or not it's about their cholesterol or heart. They are having a consultation and are given the opportunity to have a cholesterol test as well. This approach has been suggested for programmes in several countries, although the costs and benefits have yet to be fully worked out.

Selective screening

The third approach is 'selective screening', in which only certain people who are known to be at increased risk of heart disease are offered the test. For example, if someone is over 40 years old, overweight or a smoker – all risk factors for heart disease – it may be sensible to have a cholesterol check. If a person has a parent, brother, sister or child with coronary heart disease, it may be wise to have the test. If someone has high blood pressure, perhaps they should also know their cholesterol. In other words, the test is best used only if there seems, on the basis of other risk factors, to be a good case for measuring someone's cholesterol. The general assumption is that nearly everyone in a typical Western nation has a relatively high cholesterol level, and only those with other risk factors for heart disease need to know precisely what their cholesterol is.

This selective approach is likely to be the most cost-effective.

What's more, it emphasises an important point. Despite all the hype about cholesterol, with tests being offered in all sorts of unlikely places, it's important to bear in mind that your blood-cholesterol level is just one of several possible risk factors for heart and arterial disease – and that all the factors should be tackled in combination if you're really going to give your heart a new start.

What does the result mean?

You're told that your cholesterol level, say, is 6.3 or 7.2. What does that mean exactly? Before deciding on its significance, let's see what level is regarded as ideal or desirable.

A logical answer might be the average level throughout the nation. Surely, you might argue, if most other people's blood cholesterol is around a particular level, then, because it is the normal level, it must be OK, mustn't it?

Well . . . no. We've seen how closely the average cholesterol level in various countries is linked to their heart-
disease rate. Therefore, if the whole population has a
relatively high risk of heart disease by international stand-
ards (see page 33), the average blood-cholesterol level
must also be too high.

So, what level is desirable? And at what point does it
become 'raised' or 'high'?

These are obviously extremely important distinctions
because the action that people, or their doctors, need to
take depends on which category of cholesterol level
applies to them.

Dividing-lines

A number of expert committees have looked into this
matter of drawing useful dividing-lines between different
cholesterol levels and, whilst each committee has differed
slightly in its recommendations, there has been broad
agreement on what they should be. The United States
National Institutes of Health, the United States National
Cholesterol Education Program, the British Cardiac
Society, the British Hyperlipidaemia Association, the
Canadian Consensus Conference on Cholesterol and the
European Atherosclerosis Society have all set down
broadly similar dividing-lines.

Blood-cholesterol levels are usually measured not in
ounces per pint, nor even grams per litre, but in millimoles
per litre of plasma – abbreviated to 'mmol/l'. What on
earth is a millimole? Well, it's one-thousandth of the
molecular weight of cholesterol in grams. In the United
States, and occasionally elsewhere, levels are still expressed
as milligrams per decilitre (mg/dl). To convert from mg/
dl to mmol/l, you'll need to divide by 39.

The lower the figure, the better for your heart and

arteries. The risk rises fairly steadily with increasing cholesterol levels.

Less than 5.2 mmol/l (200 mg/dl): Desirable
5.2–6.4 mmol/l (200–250 mg/dl): Slightly raised
6.5–7.8 mmol/l (250–300 mg/dl): High
Over 7.8 mmol/l (300 mg/dl or more): Very high

However, the significance of an individual's cholesterol level depends very much on his or her other risk factors.

What's my risk of heart disease?

This, after all, is the crunch question for most of us. We've taken a look at ourselves, or the doctor or nurse has done it for us – our weight, our eating, exercising, smoking and drinking habits, our blood pressure and, perhaps, cholesterol and our family or personal history of heart disease – and found a long list of factors for and against. How can we assess our overall risk of premature heart trouble?

Prediction v. probability

What happens to the average person – even the average person of your age, sex, weight, fitness level, eating and smoking habits, family history and so on – will not necessarily happen to you. The effect of unknown factors that are peculiar to you and you alone must be taken into account. And, of course, there's always chance.

No amount of calculating can accurately predict what will happen to you if you do, or don't, change this or that risk factor. Assessing your risk in the sense of making a personal *prediction* is out. Some people have dreadful risk factors, but never get heart disease – others lead an exemplary life, only to succumb to a heart attack in middle age.

But that doesn't mean that estimating our risk in terms

of *probability* is not possible. It is – providing you realise that it can be nothing more than a 'best guess', based on what we know about the average effects of various risk factors among groups of people.

Rival scores

The other proviso is that any calculation of your overall heart-risk score depends entirely on which risk factors are used and how much statistical 'weight' they are given.

There have been many different attempts by experts to develop heart-risk scoring systems, using different risk factors and applying different weightings or quotients to them, in order to calculate risk scores which are both valid and useful. If too few factors are taken into account, the score lacks validity. Too many, and it becomes unwieldy.

The BRHS score

This scoring system has been derived by Professor A. G. Shaper and colleagues at the Royal Free Hospital School of Medicine in London, and is based on data from the British Regional Heart Study. It's designed for use in general practice by the doctor or practice nurse, and is only suitable for men aged 40–60 years. The purpose is to identify men who are at 'high risk' – which this particular scoring system defines as those who have a more than 50:50 chance of suffering a heart attack within five years.

The BRHS score is calculated as follows:

Number of years smoking cigarettes × 7.5
+ 4.5 × the systolic (upper) blood pressure
+ 265 if the man can recall being diagnosed as having coronary heart disease of some sort
+ 150 if the man currently has angina
+ 150 if he's diabetic
+ 80 if one of his parents died of 'heart trouble'

If a man aged 40–60 scores 1000 or more by this method he is in the 'high risk' group and should, if possible, have his blood cholesterol measured. He should also receive lifestyle advice, along the lines given later in this book, and be followed up regularly by the doctor or nurse.

You may have noticed that the BRHS score itself does not include a blood-cholesterol measurement. This is not because the blood-cholesterol level isn't important – it certainly is. But, because we know that the average middle-aged man in a Western country such as Britain has a cholesterol level that at least doubles his risk of heart disease, this assumption has already been built into the calculation. Knowing the true cholesterol in each individual case makes little difference to the final score.

What about women?

In Western countries such as Britain, women have a lower risk of heart disease than men, especially under the age of about 50. But after the menopause their risk rises quite sharply as the years go by, catching up with the male risk at about the age of 80.

The BRHS score, although not strictly appropriate for women, could be applied to those over the age of 60 as a very approximate assessment of their risk.

The Dundee score

This score, based on a survey of 10 000 typical Scots aged 40–59, can be applied to men or women. It was developed by Professor Hugh Tunstall-Pedoe and colleagues of the Cardiovascular Epidemiology Unit at the University of Dundee. Unlike the BRHS score, it makes use of the blood-cholesterol level (or, if this is not known, an estimate based on the person's age and sex). The smoking measure is also different from the BRHS score. Instead of the number of years the person has been a smoker, it uses the number of cigarettes they currently smoke daily. For blood pressure, either the systolic (upper reading) or diastolic (lower reading) can be used.

Unfortunately, the actual calculations involved are too complex to outline in this book. They are intended to be carried out by a doctor or nurse using either a simple plastic calculator, rather like a circular slide-rule, or a special computer programme.

Swings and roundabouts

The important point is that your cholesterol level, however accurately it is measured, does not mean very much on its own. Two people with the same level of cholesterol will have very different overall risks of heart disease if their other risk factors – age, sex, family history, blood pressure, smoking – differ considerably. For example, the additional risk attached to having a cholesterol over 6.5 mmol/l if you're a non-smoking man aged 35–45, with low blood pressure, may be very low indeed. But this level would add considerably to the risk of a 60-year-old male smoker with high blood pressure. These other risk factors multiply the cholesterol effect considerably.

Cholesterol in perspective

Your other heart-risk factors are the most important ones to know about – because they make the real difference in terms of your overall risk. They put your blood-cholesterol level in perspective.

If you score low on overall risk, your blood-cholesterol level is probably not worth knowing about. It would be simplest for you to assume that it's hovering around the average level for a Western nation like Britain (about 6.0 mmol/l) – and that, because this is rather higher than the desirable level, your best course of action is to change to the sort of healthier diet outlined in Chapter 8.

But if your overall risk is high, your blood-cholesterol level could be crucial, and should be measured accurately. What's more, you should look very hard at your lifestyle to see what particular risk factor, or factors, you can do something about. The next chapter will help you give your heart a new start.

— 7 —

A New Start for Your Heart

By now, you can't have failed to get the message that your overall risk of heart or arterial disease depends on a whole gamut of different risk factors, of which your blood cholesterol is but one.

Unfortunately, some you can do nothing about – your age, your sex and your family history, for instance. But if these count against you, you can at least make a special effort with the other risk factors – the ones you *can* change for the better – your eating habits, your body weight, the amount of exercise you get, your smoking and drinking habits and the way you cope with stress.

Everyone – yes, even children – should ask themselves these simple questions:

* Am I eating a healthy balance of foods?

* Am I overweight?

* Am I getting enough exercise?

* Am I hooked on smoking?

* Am I overdoing the drink?

* Am I a victim of stress?

These are the big six. To which some doctors would add, for people over 35:

* Am I getting a regular health check?

The North Karelia Project

North Karelia is the eastern part of Finland – a land of lakes, fir forests and dairy farms, bordering on Russia. In the 1960s, the people of this quiet county were found to have the highest rate of heart disease in the world. Somewhat alarmed at this revelation, and stirred into action by public health doctors, they petitioned the government to do something about it.

The result was a county-wide community campaign, started in 1972, involving television, radio, newspapers, schools, factories, shops and health centres. The aim was to reduce the main risk factors for heart disease and strokes by promoting healthy eating, helping people to stop smoking and encouraging regular blood-pressure checks.

Within 10 years, this aim had been largely achieved, especially as far as smoking was concerned, and the death rate from heart disease, particularly for men, had fallen markedly compared with the neighbouring county.

The project is continuing, and saving thousands of lives.

We shall be dealing with the whole glorious business of healthy eating in the next chapter – and giving you plenty of practical advice.

This chapter looks at the other aspects of your lifestyle which may be playing Russian roulette with your heart – to help you give it a new start.

Keeping your weight down

In Chapter 3, we looked at the effect of being overweight on your risk of heart disease and saw how it can put up your blood pressure and blood cholesterol. Apart from these concerns, obesity (being markedly overweight) is also linked to a long list of other health problems, ranging from diabetes and gallstones, to back-ache and foot problems.

We all know it's unhealthy – and yet, according to recent surveys, fatness has never been more popular. In Britain, for example, four out of 10 men, and about three out of 10 women, are overweight. In some other developed countries – notably the United States, Australia and Germany – the proportion of fatties is even higher.

Why is that? Why, despite a multi-billion-dollar slimming industry, pushing every conceivable diet, exercise machine and magic potion, are so many of us so fat? And getting fatter.

It's almost certainly because going on a 'diet', or having any other body-shaping treatment, misses the point completely. We should forget about all those persuasive pseudo-scientific explanations that accompany every latest wonder diet, and simply think about what is natural to the human body.

We evolved, an awfully long time ago, as hunter-gatherers in the great grasslands of East Africa – a species of intelligent primate, using our feet to walk and run and our hands to throw spears, set traps and gather roots, shoots and fruits. Our diet was a mixture of different foods – mostly of plant origin, but with an occasional meat treat if we got lucky. Some of us who lived near rivers, lakes or seas also ate fish and shellfish.

It was a diet largely of fibre-rich starchy foods which provided most of the bulk and energy we needed. Most of the fat and protein was also from plants, supplemented by some from animals or fish. Obtaining this food was a full-time job during the daylight hours (only 12 hours in the tropics) – so it meant a lot of walking, running, fetching and carrying. Every calorie gained took a lot of effort. Life was hard – and, of course, it still is for most of the world's population.

Nowadays, in the Western world, we've gone unbelievably soft – unhealthily comfortable. The average person's diet is light-years away from the one we were designed to eat. And the only hunting and gathering most of us do is in search of the nearest take-away!

The result is that we are suffering an epidemic of obesity the like of which we've never seen before, and we're plagued with the ultimate disease of affluence: premature coronary heart disease.

How fat is fat?

Most people who are overweight know about it – although they may not be prepared to admit it to themselves. Certainly, if you're a woman, the chances are you've been on a diet of some sort at some time in your life. Many men, too, alarmed at their middle-age spread or pot belly, make a token effort to cut down on fried breakfasts or go without the odd pint or two.

Appearances are important for most people – no one wants to look a frump or a slob. But how overweight are you as far as your health is concerned?

The chart opposite gives you the answer – and you may be surprised to find that, in health terms, you're allowed to be a little fuller in the figure than current fashion dictates.

Underweight

Are you eating enough? Eat more of the healthy balance of foods outlined in the next chapter.

If dieting is ruling your life, or you're hooked on laxatives or slimming pills, or you deliberately bring food back up after meals, you have an eating disorder which probably needs medical attention.

OK

Congratulations – you're in the optimum weight range for your health. But you may still be eating an unhealthy bal-

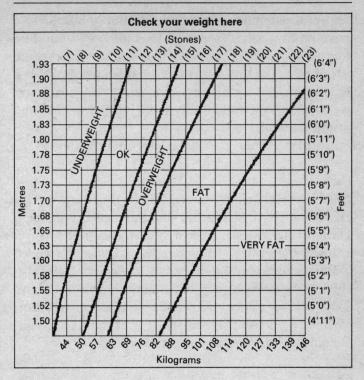

Check your weight here

Weigh yourself without clothes, and measure your height without shoes. Then check yourself against the chart: run your finger up from your weight to a point level with your height, and read off which band you're in.

ance of foods in other respects – particularly the proportions of saturated fat and fibre. Turn to the guidelines in the next chapter.

Overweight
You would do well to lose some weight, but you don't need to rush at it. No crash dieting, please – it's not at all a healthy way to stay slim. The way to tackle this moderate

degree of plumpness is not to 'diet', but to change to a more healthy balance of everyday eating, and build up your activity level a little. You'll lose weight steadily, at the rate of about 0.5 kg (1 lb) a week – in other words, about 6 kg (just under 1 stone) in 3 months. It may not sound much, but it's slow and steady and, unlike most diets, the weight stays off.

Again, there's advice for you later on in this book.

Fat

You have a real weight problem (Grade II obesity) and it's likely to affect your health if you don't get any slimmer. The most effective way to shed this extra body fat is to lose it slowly and steadily – no more than 1 kg (2 lb) a week.

This means following the healthy eating principles outlined in the next chapter, but aiming to consume about 500–750 *fewer* calories a day than you do at the moment. Not too huge a sacrifice, perhaps – but it should be enough to send your weight into a steady descent.

Very fat

You are seriously obese (Grade III obesity) and you urgently need to lose weight because it's almost certainly damaging your health. The chances are that you're only too well aware of this, and have already sought the help of a doctor. But if not, you really ought to do so – sooner rather than later.

In the meantime, use the principles outlined in the next chapter to lose no more than 1 kg (2 lb) a week by consuming up to 750 calories a day *less than you do at present*.

Pacing yourself

The starting-point for the healthy eating approach to weight loss is to give yourself plenty of time. A staggering

95 per cent of dieters fail because they try to lose too much weight too quickly. They either give up the struggle half-way through, or put the kilograms they shed straight back on again as soon as they stop the diet.

The will-power you need to lose weight successfully is not so much the will-power to help you fight the temptation of a chocolate bar or a cream cake – although that can be tough enough – but the will-power to help you fight the temptation to go on a strict diet. Strict, rigid, regimented diets may make you feel safer: the rules are 'there to be obeyed', and you probably feel you can trust yourself to stick to them simply because they are so precisely laid down. But this only works up to a point – and then it all collapses. And the reason why it collapses is that dieting isn't living.

So you must adapt your will-power to change to a healthier balance of eating, in which the key nutrients are in balance with each other, and the calorie content is in balance with the energy requirements of your lifestyle. That way, the weight you lose will stay lost. And the benefits of being slimmer will be lasting.

Getting more exercise

Not only is regular exercise a useful way to help you burn up calories, and hence lose weight, it also has a number of other beneficial effects that help to reduce your risk of heart disease.

It increases your HDL level. This, you'll remember, is the 'protective' lipoprotein that helps to remove harmful cholesterol from your arteries.

It helps to reduce raised blood pressure. Although your blood pressure naturally rises during a bout of exercise or any physical exertion, in order to force more blood to the working muscles, regular exercise has been shown to lower

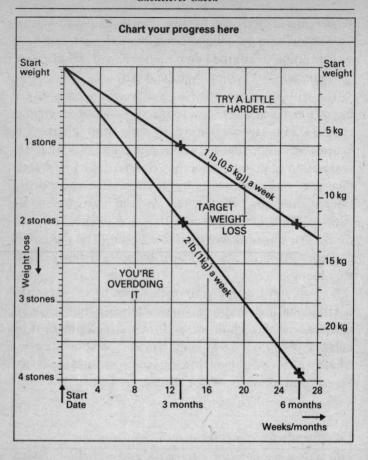

Chart your progress here

Start weight — TRY A LITTLE HARDER — Start weight

1 lb (0.5 kg)) a week

TARGET WEIGHT LOSS

2 lb (1kg) a week

YOU'RE OVERDOING IT

Weight loss ↓

1 stone — 5 kg
2 stones — 10 kg
3 stones — 15 kg
4 stones — 20 kg

Start Date — 4 — 8 — 12 — 16 — 20 — 24 — 28
3 months — 6 months

Weeks/months →

Mark your present weight with a cross on the left-hand scale, and put today's date (or whenever you want to start) at the left-hand end of the time-scale along the bottom. Assuming a weight loss of about 0.5 kg (1 lb) a week, mark a cross 6 kg (about 1 stone) lighter in 3 months' time, and another 12 kg (nearly 2 stone) lighter in 6 months' time. Join the two crosses with a line. Now do the same thing assuming a weight loss of 1 kg (2 lb) a week, and draw another line.

Weigh yourself weekly (not more often – it's demoralising!) at about the same time of day and enter your weight on the chart. You should aim to keep your weekly progress within the two lines.

the *resting* blood-pressure level. This is the blood pressure at rest, between periods of exercise – which, for most people, is most of the time.

It's a useful way to combat stress. Research has found that regular, non-competitive, rhythmic, aerobic activity – such as walking, running, swimming, dancing, skipping or cycling – helps to reduce adrenalin and noradrenalin ('stress hormone') levels in the circulation, and stimulate endorphin ('pleasure hormone') levels in the brain. It has been successfully used by psychiatrists in Britain, Scandinavia and America to treat severe anxiety and depression.

And last but not least, many smokers find that, by taking up a more active lifestyle, it's easier for them to really commit themselves to giving up the weed – and to succeed.

All in all, as we found in Chapter 3, by adopting a moderately active lifestyle, with a fair amount of aerobic activity each week, we can reduce our risk of a heart attack *by up to a half*.

So, the case for regular exercise – for your heart's sake – is impressive. Here are the plus-points again:

Regular aerobic exercise:

✴ Helps you to lose weight and stay slim

✴ Helps to increase the 'protective' HDL in your blood

✴ Helps to reduce high blood pressure

✴ Helps to combat stress

✴ And all this in addition to improving your stamina, suppleness and strength.

What is 'aerobic' activity?

This doesn't just mean the type of exercises known as 'aerobics' – although they are certainly included in a long list of activities that are aerobic.

Aerobic activity is any activity that increases your breathing rate – making you slightly, or not so slightly, puffed. Here are the main basic aerobic activities:

* Walking, the brisker the better

* Jogging, comfortably and enjoyably

* 'Jarming', arm-jogging for chairbound people

* Swimming, doing lengths when the pool is quiet

* Cycling, indoors or out, good for arthritis

* Skipping, try it to music

* Dancing, definitely better to music

* Exercising on the spot (for example, aerobics), with or without music

Aerobic activities involve the rhythmic, dynamic contraction of large muscle groups – especially the legs. The constantly working muscles demand more oxygen from the bloodstream, and you breathe harder to replace it.

What about sports and games?

Most sports and games have a worthwhile aerobic component to them. The few exceptions include such exertions as weightlifting and wrestling, which involve more isometric (straining) activity. Isometrics push up the blood pressure and are definitely not to be recommended as a healthy way to help your heart, especially if you're an older person (over 45!).

Older people would be wise also to avoid fiercely competitive, vigorous sports, such as squash or football, unless they are already fit. These sports tend to involve rapid bursts of activity, coupled with a high degree of alertness or aggression, and the combined effect is to increase adrenalin/noradrenalin levels, blood pressure, pulse rate, cholesterol level and the 'irritability' of the heart muscle.

So choose steadier forms of exertion, that involve the sorts of rhythmic activities mentioned above.

It's crucial to find something you enjoy doing. It's absolutely no good at all if you embark on a punishing schedule of work-outs or gym-bashing that gets you fighting fit in 6 weeks, but is too gruelling to keep up for much longer than that.

Rather like crash dieting, there's no mileage in power-training – at least, not for your heart. The benefits of an active lifestyle pay dividends over decades, not just between now and your next seaside holiday!

How much, and how often?

The generally recommended advice, for a relatively unfit person, is to start very gently and build up very gradually – just push yourself enough to get a little short of breath. Not gasping – but definitely breathing hard. Aim for a level of exertion you can keep up continuously for about 20 minutes at a time, with no more than a few brief breaks.

For most people, this will mean little more than the equivalent of brisk walking to start with. But as your fitness gradually improves over the next few weeks, you can start to do a little more each time.

You'll need at least three of these 20-minute (or thereabouts) periods of aerobic activity more or less every week, in order to derive a useful benefit for your heart. But less

Benefits of activities			
	Stamina	Strength	Suppleness
Jogging, medium	★★	★	★
Running	★★★	★	★
Cycling, hard	★★★	★★	★
Rowing	★★★	★★	★
Swimming, hard	★★★	★★	★★
Dancing, hard aerobic	★★★	★★	★★★
Walking, brisk	★★	★	★
Soccer	★★	★	★
Dancing, hard disco	★★	★	★★
Badminton	★★	★	★★★
Squash	★★★	★	★★★
Tennis	★	★	★★
Weight lifting	★	★★★	★
Judo	★	★★	★★
Golf	★	★	★

★★★ = very good ★★ = effective ★ = little effect

than that certainly helps most people, and you don't need to stick to a rigid schedule.

How safe is exercise?

Bearing in mind the provisos about isometrics and vigorous competitive sports, and about starting gently and building up gradually, you needn't worry that exercise might be dangerous. As long as you choose the right sort of activity, don't push yourself too hard and never do anything that's even uncomfortable, let alone painful, you'll enjoy its benefits without injuring yourself.

The scientific evidence shows that it's far safer to be physically active, or a regular exerciser, than to be inactive or sedentary. Even for people with existing heart disease, a sensible, steady approach to exercise is beneficial because it improves the coronary circulation.

The sort of person who comes unstuck with exercise is the middle-aged sedentary male, usually a thrusting executive type, anxious to get fit quick, who throws himself hammer and tongs into a 'needle' game like squash, thrashes his opponent around the court, and then wonders why he's pulled a muscle or feels giddy.

Exercise is for life – not to prove something to yourself or others. It's best if it becomes part of your everyday existence, rather than a 'programme' or 'regime' or 'prescription' that you have to force yourself into.

Is a medical check-up necessary?

Most people, even older people, don't need a medical check-up before they move to a more active lifestyle. But it may be best to have a word with your doctor if you suffer from one of the following conditions:

✳ high blood pressure or heart disease

✳ a chronic chest problem like asthma or bronchitis

✳ back trouble or a slipped disc

✳ joint pains or arthritis

✳ diabetes

✳ any other condition you think might be affected

✳ . . . or if you're recovering from a recent illness or operation

In fact, exercise of the right sort can be good for all these conditions. However, it may affect the treatment you're being given, and your doctor ought really to have a chance to discuss it with you.

Everyday activity

Try to 'think physical', and look for ways to increase your activity every day – to burn up more calories and make more use of your body. Here are some examples:

* Use the stairs more often, up as well as down

* Get off the bus a stop or two sooner

* Surprise your dog, walk faster and further

* Play more active games with your children

* Use weekends to get out and about, on your feet

Final thoughts

As far as your heart and arteries are concerned, the important thing about exercise is that it should become so much a natural part of your life that it makes you feel good, and you miss it if you can't get it.

Remember the three Fs: Activity should be Fun, Frequent and Fizzical!

Giving up smoking

In Chapter 3 we saw how cigarette smoking can double your risk of heart disease by:

* constricting arteries

* interfering with blood lipids

* spoiling the oxygen-carrying efficiency of blood

* making blood more likely to clot

* . . . and a number of other unpleasantries

Combined with a high cholesterol, your risk is multiplied even more.

Survey after survey shows that more and more smokers really want to give up. Or rather, they do and they don't. They would like to have given up, to be non-smokers. But they don't like the idea of going through the process of giving up – the fear of 'cold turkey'.

If you're one of these 'floating smokers', hovering on the brink of stopping, let's hope this book will help you take the plunge.

If you're a confirmed smoker, and resent any attempt to persuade you otherwise, or are convinced that it's too late to change now, please go back and look through the evidence again. See for yourself, and decide for yourself.

Yes – but how?
The chances are you've tried giving up before – perhaps more times than you care to remember. But were you *really* determined to succeed? Did you have enough encouragement and support? Did you have a method, or did you just throw yourself into it?

There's no question that nicotine is a highly addictive drug. Although it lacks the euphoric effect of heroin, its ability to 'hook' the user is not so very different. If cigarettes had been introduced on to the streets today, they would have been banned immediately.

This means that many hardened smokers find it very difficult to give up. For them, 'cold turkey' is too much to bear. The relief at finally capitulating, and having that much-craved-for cigarette, is overwhelming. It puts them back on the rails again – and they give up giving up. This is a tragedy as far as their health is concerned, because it's these heavy smokers who have most to gain from stopping.

But for most smokers (less than 20 a day), giving up

needn't be as traumatic as this. If you're a smoker you'll know how long you can go without a cigarette. You'll know that it depends on what you're doing, who you're with and where you are. You may even have found out that you can go all day without a cigarette, and not miss it.

Much of the smoking habit is just that: habit. You've got used to doing it at particular times of day or in particular places – perhaps with your coffee, when you're on the telephone, if you're waiting somewhere, in the car, during tea breaks, at the pub, watching television . . . You find yourself in a 'trigger' situation, or doing a 'trigger' activity, and – ping! – a bell rings in your subconscious and you reach for your cigarettes. Pure Pavlov.

So, to win at giving up smoking, you may have to overcome two hurdles, depending on what kind of smoker you are. If nicotine is important to you, you'll have to shake off your physical and psychological dependence on it. And if you're locked into the ritual of smoking, you'll have to find ways of breaking the cycle. If, like most smokers, you fall into both camps, you'll need an approach to giving up that deals with both dependence and habit.

If all this is putting you off the idea, remember you're not alone. Millions of people have succeeded.

Steps to success
We haven't room to go into a full programme for giving up smoking, but here are a few steps in the process.

1 Make the decision and stick to it
This is the absolutely crucial step. Unless you're convinced you want to give up, and that this is the time you're really going to do it, you won't stand a chance. No one can give up for you. Of course, other people can help by being supportive, taking your mind off cigarettes and keeping

you on an even keel. But when it comes down to it, only you (the real, deep-down, inner you) can make the decision to go for it.

Re-think all the reasons why you should give up. Write them down, and put them in priority order. Think how your life will change when you're a non-smoker. Write down a list of the benefits.

Try to persuade a friend, your partner or a workmate to give up with you. Apart from the fact that it's very difficult to stop smoking if someone close to you is carrying on with it, you can do a lot to help each other win through.

2 Prepare to stop

You're probably dreading the oncoming battle with yourself. Despite going through Step 1, you're bound to be in two minds about giving up. Part of you has made the firm decision – and the other will do anything for a cigarette. So, like any battle, it's won or lost in the preparation.

Name a date to give up in about 1 week's time (maybe 2 if life is a bit hectic at the moment). It's best to pick a day which is fairly typical, in the sense that as far as you know you won't be under any particular pressure or additional stress. It may be an ordinary working day – say a Monday – or a Saturday or Sunday when you're relaxing.

Tell your friends and colleagues (especially the non-smokers) about your decision, and which day you'll be stopping. It will help to reinforce your determination. You won't want to let yourself down.

Buy a cheap little notebook and keep a 'smoking diary' for the week or so before you stop. It's not too much effort. All you have to do is make a note of the day and time when you have a cigarette, what you were doing, who you were with and how much you needed it (a little, a lot, somewhere in between?). Write this down before you light up, to make sure you get the facts right.

Try to cut down the number of cigarettes you smoke. Look at your smoking diary and see which ones you could have done without. Try to miss them next time. One trick is to put a rubber band round the packet so that you have to think twice about each cigarette – do I really need this one right now? Another is to put the pack in a less accessible place. Yet another is not to carry matches or a lighter, so that you have to keep asking for a light.

Keep two jam jars. In one, put as many of your cigarette-ends as you can muster, adding to your collection as you go along. At the end of each day, have a good look and a good sniff. In the other, collect exactly the same amount of money as you spend on cigarettes. Put it in before you buy each packet. At the end of the week, compare the two jars. When you give up, keep filling the money jar – it's your ever-growing jackpot.

3 The day you stop

The moment you wake up, tell yourself you're now a non-smoker. Make the mental leap. Try to convince yourself that, rather than being a smoker who is not going to smoke, you're a non-smoker who doesn't need to smoke. True, you're only a beginner at non-smoking (or shall we say 'out of practice'?) and you may have some difficulty to start with. But basically, you are a natural non-smoker and you won't need to put any cigarettes in your mouth today.

Aim just to get through this one day without having a cigarette. Don't contemplate the next 2 or 3 weeks of 'pain and anguish'. Take one day at a time.

Remove all cigarettes, lighters, ashtrays and other smoking paraphernalia from your presence. Perhaps even make a ceremony of it – the casting out of the evil weed!

Check your smoking diary, and try to find ways of avoiding the situations in which you really needed a cigarette. For example, you could have an orange juice or munch an apple instead of having coffee. You could have a sandwich in the park instead of going to the pub or the cafeteria. You could chew some sugar-free gum when you're on the telephone or in a tense situation. You could have a sugar-free mint after lunch or supper. Think of ways you can break the ritual. Find diversions and distractions. You may feel a bit isolated, or even silly at times, but persevere – this battle is too important to be taken lightly.

If you get an overwhelming craving in a tight spot, or find yourself becoming unbearably tense, try deep breathing. Breathe in slowly and quietly all the way, filling every corner of your lungs with air – and then, equally slowly and quietly, let your breath out in a long, smoothly controlled expiration until your lungs are completely empty. Repeat this, over and over again, until the craving subsides.

4 Staying stopped

Remember to take just one day at a time – make a determined effort to get through it without a cigarette. Look again at your list of reasons for stopping. Look again at your jam-jar jackpot.

Develop new habits to replace smoking. Things to chew or munch (preferably non-fattening), things to do with your hands, fresh-tasting drinks instead of tea or coffee, new places to go in your breaks.

If you're worried about putting on weight (by no means always a problem), surround yourself with low-calorie comforters – mineral water, low-calorie drinks, sugar-free gum, apples, tangerines, carrots and many others. Weight gain after giving up smoking is usually temporary, whilst your metabolism readjusts to the absence of nicotine. After 2 or 3 weeks, you'll start to shed it again, providing you don't overload yourself with calories.

Keep on your guard. It's very tempting after a week or two, or even 6 months, to tell yourself you can take it or leave it, and that you will allow yourself just one cigarette as a reward for all your self-denial (. . . why not?).

Oh, frailty! This is the classic error. This is what happens to so many people who do so well to get so far – only to stumble at the last fence.

This does not mean that the whole effort is wasted if you do succumb to a cigarette. It isn't – if you can put that moment of weakness behind you and carry on where you left off. But, by accepting that one cigarette, you make it much harder for yourself not to accept another, and another, and then to buy a packet for yourself. You know the story – you've probably been through it already.

So keep on being a non-smoker who doesn't need a cigarette. Day after day after day, it gets easier and easier.

Tips for heavy smokers

✳ Spend more time, about 3 or 4 weeks, preparing to give up by gradually cutting down the number of cigarettes you smoke. Use the smoking-diary method outlined above to decide which cigarettes you can most easily do without. Switch to a lower-tar brand, and smoke less of each cigarette. This way you can cut down your dependence on nicotine so that, when you do finally take the plunge, it won't be so difficult.

✳ You may find that carrying a packet containing just one cigarette, for emergency use only, is enough of a safety net to see you through each day. That's fine – as long as you never smoke it, except under the direst of circumstances.

✳ Another method is to start substituting nicotine-containing chewing gum for cigarettes, so that on the day you give up you can keep your blood level of nicotine high enough to avoid the worst cravings. You'll still need to use all the dodges outlined above to break the mechanical ritual of lighting up, but over the next few weeks these urges will subside and you can slowly wean yourself off the gum.

✳ Many heavy or dependent smokers are greatly helped by hypnosis or acupuncture. The former can be a very effective way of tackling the problem of will-power – but does not work so well for everybody. The latter helps to combat the physical discomfort of nicotine withdrawal – and again is not suitable for everyone.

✳ There are several good books on ways to give up smoking. If you'd like professional help, your doctor should be able to advise you or point you in the direction of a stop-smoking group or a suitable course.

Coping with stress

It's tempting to blame stress for almost every ill. Certainly, our image of the classic heart-attack or stroke victim is someone who is under pressure, flustered, overdoing things or getting too hot under the collar.

We have already seen that, although tension and anxiety can raise blood-cholesterol levels, it is difficult to prove the links between stress and heart disease or stroke, or even to know exactly what stress is and how to measure it.

Nevertheless, most of us recognise stress when we're suffering it. We usually know when things are getting on top of us, or when we're getting far too tense. And if we don't recognise it in ourselves, other people usually spot the signs and symptoms pretty early on.

An inability to relax, constant anxiety, grinding teeth, white knuckles, poor sleep, too much smoking or drinking, perhaps over-eating, skin troubles, bowel disturbances . . . the list goes on and on.

Obviously, your personality has a lot to do with the way

you cope with stressful situations – one person's stress is another person's stimulation. You may thrive on huge responsibilities or constant deadlines. You may love unrelenting pressure. People in positions of authority tend to thrive on 'stress'; it is often those who have less control who suffer more.

But most of us can do without too much adrenalin surging round our systems. We need to find ways to combat or avoid the ravages of stress.

In this section, we look at a few simple techniques for helping ourselves to relax and keep stress at bay.

Crisis? – what crisis?

The first step is to recognise that stress may be playing rather a large part in your life. It means asking yourself a few very fundamental questions, such as:

✳ What are the most important things in my life? My family? My friends? My job? My hobbies? My health?

✳ How much time do I have to give to my real priorities?

✳ How much time do I have for myself?

✳ How can I manage my time better?

✳ How can I parcel out my tasks more efficiently?

✳ Do I really need to do everything I think I need to do?

✳ Can I be more realistic about what I can sensibly take on, and what I can't?

✳ Can I find someone else to help shoulder my burdens?

You may find that by standing back for a moment and reappraising your life and the way you run it, or it runs you, you can make a few adjustments that pay huge dividends in reducing stress. Of course, many of us have such major worries – about money, job (or lack of it), relationships, neighbours – that there may seem to be no easy answers. But usually, by thinking about as many options as you can and, better still, by talking them over with someone you know well and can trust, you'll find that solutions begin to present themselves. Light starts to appear at the end of the tunnel. Your crisis begins to resolve itself.

Stressful moments

Even if your life is reasonably under control, there are bound to be moments which are a little, or a lot, too stressful for comfort. It might be an important meeting, an emotional occasion, all the children shouting at once, a traffic jam, a family row – the list is endless. Or it might be the culmination of a particularly tough day or week, or the few awful days before your period.

Whatever the cause, there are ways in which you can use your mind and your body to ease away tension, and reduce anxiety. In short, you can learn to relax.

Relaxation techniques

There are many different approaches, but they all use the body to calm the mind, or the mind to relax the body.

✷ *Deep breathing*

When you're tense you take rapid, shallow breaths through your mouth. By breathing slowly and deeply through your nose, you can ease away tension.

Sit comfortably in a chair, preferably in a quiet room, with your eyes shut. Start by taking in a very long, steady breath, right into every corner of your lungs. Hold it for a few seconds and then let it out very slowly, all of it, without forcing it. Just relax, and let the air flow out under its own momentum. Hold your lungs empty for a few seconds and then breathe in again.

As you repeat this, think about nothing but your breathing. Then, once you're into a slow, steady rhythm, picture waves breaking on a shingle beach so that the sound of your breathing becomes the ebb and flow of the sea.

✳ *Progressive relaxation*
This is a way of relaxing groups of muscles, one by one.

Sit comfortably in a chair, preferably in a quiet room, with your eyes shut. Now think about your feet – concentrate on relaxing them, letting them feel heavy, so heavy that they want to sink through the floor. Next, focus on your legs. Let the tension drain out of them, let the muscles relax, let your thighs drift apart if they want to. Now concentrate on your trunk. Let your tummy drift in and out with your quiet breathing. Next, your hands and arms. Let them feel as though they're made of lead, heavy and immobile. And your shoulders, totally relaxed, no tension at all. Balance your head on your neck, relax your cheeks and finally unknit your brow and imagine soft fingers stroking your forehead.

✳ *Meditation*
Don't be put off by preconceived ideas about flower power or psychedelia. Meditation has been practised for centuries, especially in the Orient, and is a remarkable way of achieving inner calm. It takes deep breathing and progressive relaxation a stage further.

Sit comfortably in a chair, preferably in a quiet room, with your eyes shut. After a minute or so of deep breathing, and relaxing yourself from your feet upwards, focus your mind's eye on a point *between* your two eyes (keeping them shut). Think of it as a tunnel. Now let the tunnel draw your thoughts into itself, as though it were sucking all your worries and tensions into the far distance. This is difficult to explain, but once it starts to happen you'll know the feeling. All your thoughts are focused on the tunnel, all distractions are sucked into it, and your head becomes wonderfully uncluttered.

After a few minutes of this, you can allow yourself to open your eyes and 'snap out of it'. If you're doing it right, you'll find you feel greatly refreshed.

✳ *Rhythmic exercise*
The benefits of rhythmic aerobic exercise were described on page 93.

There's no doubt that activities like walking, running, swimming, skipping, dancing or cycling are all very good ways of easing away tension – provided you find a hassle-free time and place for them. Cycling to work in heavy traffic is hardly relaxing. Neither is trying to do lengths in a crowded swimming pool.

Obviously, the big advantage of exercise as a way of letting off steam is that it has many other health benefits.

✳ *Warm baths, soft music, massage, sex, yoga*
These are just a few of the many other ways you could relax in your spare time – in no particular order!

What is important is to make sure you give yourself enough time to unwind, even if it's only a few minutes each day.

Blood pressure
In Chapter 3 we saw how a high blood pressure can multiply the damaging effect of a high cholesterol and so increase your risk of heart disease or a stroke. But what is high blood pressure, and what can you do about it?

Absolutely vital

The term 'blood pressure' refers to the pressure of the blood in your main arteries (blood in veins is under virtually no pressure, apart from the effect of gravity and the action of nearby muscles).

The arterial blood has to be under pressure so that it can be forced through smaller and smaller branches, and then through microscopic capillaries in the tissues. If you're standing or sitting up, the pressure must also overcome gravity so that the blood reaches your brain. So blood pressure is absolutely vital.

Problems arise when it is too high or too low. Too high, and you risk heart disease, a stroke and kidney trouble. Too low, and you pass out in a faint or in shock.

Constant control

Your blood pressure is under the constant control of a remarkable system of pressure detectors and adjusters. Suffice it to say that this system is incredibly complex, and we're only just beginning to unravel its mysteries.

Many factors can shift the balance. It can very quickly be pushed up by anger, excitement, exercise or pain. And it can drop as a result of fear, nausea, overheating, emotional shock, allergic reaction, haemorrhage or severe diarrhoea.

But these are immediate effects. What about long-term changes to your ordinary resting blood pressure? More to the point, what makes it rise too high?

Going up

About one adult in 10 has high blood pressure (hypertension) so, as you'd expect, the main causative factors are fairly common. They are:

* being overweight

* lack of regular exercise

✻ moderate or heavy drinking

✻ being sensitive to sodium in the diet (for example, salt)

✻ being under chronic stress

✻ having high blood pressure in the family

Less common are various medical causes – certain hormonal, metabolic and kidney disorders.

Going down

We looked at the problems of weight control and lack of exercise earlier in this chapter, and have just dealt with stress.

There's not much you can do about a family tendency to high blood pressure, apart from having yours checked regularly, and being extra careful about the other factors that may be linked to blood pressure.

That leaves alcohol and sodium. Current evidence suggests that each is likely to be an important factor for a proportion of the population, but that people who are sensitive to the hypertensive effects of alcohol are not necessarily those who are sensitive to sodium. What's more, there's no easy way at present of finding out which of us is sensitive to what.

In other words, the most sensible course of action, especially if there's high blood pressure in your family, or you already have it yourself, is to go easy on both alcohol and sodium.

Alcohol

Drink is a great social lubricant, the source of much pleasure and an easy way to relax. For most people in the developed world, life would be pretty dreary without it.

The trouble, as we all know, is that it has a 'down side'.

Apart from a long list of social problems linked to over-indulgence – from accidents to arson, and from marital bust-ups to pub punch-ups – there are several major, long-term health risks. Most people are familiar with such disorders as cirrhosis of the liver, vitamin deficiency and loss of memory brought on by chronic heavy drinking. But not so many are aware of the link between excessive drinking and high blood pressure. In fact, over-indulgence in alcohol is about twice as common among hypertensive people as it is among those with normal blood pressure.

Within limits

There are clear guidelines from most national expert bodies on the limits for sensible drinking. In Britain, for instance, the Royal College of Physicians, together with a number of other eminent organisations, has recommended the following:

✳ For men, the sensible limit is 21 units of alcohol a week.

✳ For women, the limit is 14 units of alcohol a week.

A 'unit' is: a *half* pint of ordinary beer, lager or cider (less if it's strong or extra strong)
a pub glass of table wine
a single pub measure of any spirit
a small pub schooner of sherry, port or vermouth

Remember, these are pub measures. Drinks poured out at home tend to be rather more generous.

Now, these limits may strike you as restrictive. After all, many men would regard a daily half-pint at lunch-time, and just one pint in the evening, as virtually teetotal. And just two glasses of wine a day would, for many women, be real self-denial.

And yet, for some people, any more than that and their

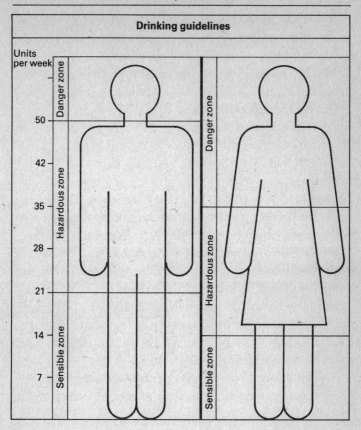

Drinking guidelines

Units per week

Danger zone
50
42
35
Hazardous zone
28
21
14
Sensible zone
7

risk of developing high blood pressure starts to rise. The danger comes with daily drinking – the more you drink every day, the higher your blood pressure is likely to creep.

Staying low
It is important to be aware of how much you're drinking. Most people never stop to think about it. They regard themselves as 'social drinkers', and so it must be OK.

It might be a sobering exercise to keep a diary of what you drink, when, where and with whom. You may surprise yourself.

If you are over the limit most of the time, you'd be wise to find ways of cutting down. Smaller tots, fewer rounds, slower sips, low- or no-alcohol alternatives.

And try to have two or three completely alcohol-free days each week. You'll be amazed how easy it is.

If it isn't, you probably need help. (There's an address at the end of the book.)

Sodium

As many as one person in four may be sensitive to sodium's effect on blood pressure – although not all these people will actually develop permanent hypertension.

Nevertheless, recent evidence gleaned from 78 dietary trials worldwide, involving 47 000 people, has led to the conclusion that eating half a teaspoon *less* a day of salt would prevent one person in five from having a premature stroke, one in six from succumbing to premature heart disease, and halve the number of people needing to take drugs to reduce their blood pressure.

Not all experts would agree with these estimates. But there is broad agreement that we should be eating much less salt.

Much less salt

The average salt consumption in a typical Western nation, such as Britain, is about 12 g (½ oz) a day. The World Health Organization recommends no more than 6 g (¼ oz) a day. In other words, on average, we should cut our salt intake by half.

To achieve this kind of reduction, we should avoid salty foods (see the table opposite), be much more sparing about adding salt in cooking and remove salt from the table. As well as that, food manufacturers should drastically reduce the amount they add in processing.

Easy does it

No doubt you're thinking that this sounds a little draconian, to say the least. Surely it can only mean that food will be utterly tasteless.

Well, surprisingly, no – not if you cut down very gradually over a few weeks. It's a matter of re-educating your taste-buds, which have become used to the high levels of salt most people consume – many times more than your body actually needs.

Salt in foods (a few examples)

Food	Sodium g/100g
High	
Grilled bacon	2.00
Sweet pickle	1.70
Canned ham	1.25
Steamed smoked haddock	1.22
Cornflakes	1.14
Tomato ketchup	1.12
Grilled pork sausages	1.00
Medium	
Brown sauce	.98
Butter (salted)	.87
Margarine	.80
Cheddar cheese	.61
Bread	.58
Crisps	.55
Salted peanuts	.44
Fish fingers	.35
Cream cheese	.30
Low	
Raw eggs	.14
Fresh steamed salmon	.11
Full cream milk	.09

Food	Sodium *g/100g*
Roast pork	.08
Roast beef	.05
Fresh fruit	.01
Negligible *(less than .01%)*	–
Fresh peanuts (unsalted)	–
Boiled potato	–
Peas	–

Medication for high blood pressure

The trouble with high blood pressure is that you don't know you've got it until something goes wrong (like a heart attack), or it's detected at a health check-up.

All adults, especially those over 35 years of age, should have their blood pressure checked at least once every 3 years. Some doctors would say more often than that.

When you have your blood pressure checked, you sit quietly in a chair or on a couch and the nurse or doctor puts an inflatable rubber cuff round your upper arm. This is connected to a pressure gauge and then inflated with air until it temporarily stops the flow of blood in your arm artery. Then the pressure is released and, as it slowly falls, two readings are taken: one when the pulse first returns to the artery (the upper or systolic pressure) and one when the flow is continuous between pulses (the lower or diastolic pressure). Thus your blood pressure is expressed as two numbers. For example:

$$120/80 \text{ mmHg}$$

(The units refer to the height in millimetres of a column of mercury that could be held up by that pressure, abbreviated to 'mmHg'.)

How high is too high?

This is a very good question, and has been the subject of much medical debate. As we saw in Chapter 3, the higher the blood pressure, the greater the risk of heart disease and strokes. So where should the line be drawn between a normal or desirable blood pressure, and one that is too high? And at what level should medication be added to the sort of self-help remedies outlined earlier in this chapter?

The answers to these questions have been decided by international committees of experts who have produced guidelines by weighing up the level of risk against the effectiveness of treatment, bearing in mind any adverse side-effects of treatment and the cost to health services. It's a complex computation, and we haven't room to go into it here, but, in general, the recommendations are that blood-pressure measurements be divided into three bands: mild, moderate and severe.

Treating high blood pressure

Mild hypertension is usually reduced by self-help methods – losing weight, cutting down on salt and alcohol, taking more exercise, learning to relax.

Moderate hypertension requires these changes in lifestyle, plus daily antihypertensive (blood pressure lowering) medication and regular check-ups.

Severe hypertension requires these changes and stronger medication, with frequent check-ups. Various tests are usually conducted to try to find a cause for the very high blood pressure.

Large-scale trials of these treatments have shown that the incidence of strokes can be greatly reduced – by well over half – and coronary heart disease cut by more than one-tenth. Kidney and eye complications of high blood pressure are also significantly reduced.

The results would be even better were it not for two disadvantages. The first is that, because the great majority of people with hypertension have no symptoms, they often fail to take their medication regularly, especially if the tablets make them feel tired (as some do). The second is that some antihypertensive drugs – particularly thiazide diuretics (urine-makers) and most beta-blockers (heart-steadiers) – tend to increase the level of blood cholesterol and triglycerides, and decrease the protective HDL. Alpha-blockers avoid these negative effects.

Newer drug treatments, without these disadvantages, are being developed. But in the meantime, if your blood pressure is raised there are three important messages:

✳ Make changes to your lifestyle to lose excess weight, cut down on salt and alcohol, take more exercise and avoid stress (outlined earlier in this chapter).

✳ Take your antihypertensive medication daily and keep your check-up appointments.

✳ Make extra efforts to keep your cholesterol down through healthy eating (see next chapter).

Cholesterol-lowering drug treatment
If you have a high cholesterol level that stays worryingly high, even after months on a low-fat, high-soluble-fibre diet, the doctor might recommend trying daily medication to help bring it down. If you have an inherited form of hyperlipidaemia, drug treatment is probably essential.

Here are the main types of medication:

Bile-acid binding resins
These work in a similar way to foods high in soluble fibre, such as oatbran and beans. The medications are artificial resins which, as with fibre, pass straight through the ali-

mentary tract without being digested or absorbed. Rather like blotting-paper, they soak up the bile which has been squirted into the intestine from the gall bladder and liver. Normally, bile acids are re-absorbed into the system a little further down the intestine, and carried back to the liver for recycling – but the resin prevents this from happening, and the bile acids are excreted. This means the liver has to make more bile, which uses up more cholesterol. In this way, the blood-cholesterol level is lowered.

There are two commonly prescribed bile binder resins: cholestyramine and colestipol. Both are rather gritty powders that have to be mixed with water or fruit juice. They are usually very effective at lowering cholesterol, by 15–30 per cent. But they can cause bowel disturbances and, because they interfere with the absorption of the fat-soluble Vitamins A, D, E and K, have to be taken with vitamin supplements.

Fibrates

These drugs probably work by interfering with the production of cholesterol and hastening the breakdown of the fatty particles in the blood, thus reducing triglycerides. They also raise beneficial HDL. There are four commonly prescribed drugs in this group: clofibrate, bezafibrate, fenofibrate and gemfibrozil. The first three usually lower cholesterol by 5–15 per cent; gemfibrozil does rather better. HDL can rise by up to about 10 per cent.

Nicotinic acid (niacin)

In small doses, up to 20 mg, nicotinic acid is a vitamin in the B group, Vitamin B3, and is widely available in such foods as wholemeal bread, wholegrain cereals, bran, nuts, pulses, yeast, meat and liver. It's involved in the metabolism of carbohydrates, and a deficiency causes the disease pellagra, virtually unheard of in the developed world.

In very high doses – mega-doses of at least 10 times the vitamin level – nicotinic acid can interfere with the production of cholesterol in the liver, lowering blood cholesterol by 10–30 per cent. It also seems to increase the level of beneficial HDL. As a food supplement, it's widely

---

Can atheroma plaques ever disappear?

During the Second World War, pathologists performing autopsies noticed that the fatty streaks and atheroma plaques they had been used to finding in dead people's arteries before the war seemed to be a thing of the past. Fewer and fewer arteries showed any evidence of them from about 1942 onwards, especially in Europe. It was the 1950s before they started to return, and over the next two decades became worse than ever. The most promising theory to explain these changes was that the lowered incidence of fatty streaks and plaques had probably been the result of food shortages and rationing, particularly of lard, meat and dairy products, during the war.

Subsequently, research on rhesus monkeys and pigs with artificially induced atherosclerosis has shown that, if they are fed on a low-fat, low-cholesterol diet for up to 4 years, the atheroma plaques in their arteries get appreciably smaller. This is interesting – but does the same apply to humans?

Human hearts

There's some evidence from controlled studies that people on a cholesterol-lowering diet, or taking cholesterol-lowering drugs, can also diminish the furring up of their arteries caused by atheroma plaques.

The studies use a technique called coronary angiography. This involves threading a catheter (a long, thin plastic tube) up a main artery, into the aorta, and thence into the opening of each coronary artery. A special dye, injected through the catheter, shows up on an X-ray, and clearly outlines the

---

available in health food shops, and can be bought over the counter in chemist shops.

So why isn't it the answer to all our prayers?

The reason is that in these huge doses it causes an unpleasant hot flush, and often an itchy rash too. What's more, we really don't know what adverse effects this might

---

plaques of atheroma as ragged constrictions.

One such study took place in Leiden in the Netherlands. A total of 39 patients with stable angina each had a coronary angiogram performed on them before being put on a strict vegetarian diet for 2 years. At the end of that period, they underwent a repeat angiogram to see what effect, if any, the diet had had on their atheroma plaques. Although the plaques had increased in 21 of the patients, there was no change in 18 of them. What's more, the patients who showed no change were those with the lowest blood cholesterols and highest HDLs. Although no one's plaques had actually 'regressed' (diminished), the study at least demonstrated that atherosclerosis can be halted.

How about drug treatment?

More recent studies have been even more encouraging. Two major regression trials in the United States, each involving larger numbers of patients than in Leiden, and each using cholesterol-lowering drugs, have also shown that atherosclerosis can be stopped in its tracks. But the real breakthrough came with a trial using a combination of the cholesterol-lowering drug colestipol and nicotinic acid. With this trial, the atheroma was not only stopped – in a significant number of plaques it was actually put into reverse. In other words, some plaques regressed a little. Not a lot, but a little.

Now even more powerful cholesterol-lowering drugs such as lovastatin, simvastatin and pravastatin are available – and trials are currently being carried out to see if they are even better at shrinking atheroma plaques.

have over a period of years – so it certainly should not be taken without consulting a doctor.

Nicotinic acid clones

The drugs in this group are derived from nicotinic acid (otherwise known as niacin or Vitamin B3). It's been known for some years that mega-doses of nicotinic acid can lower cholesterol, probably by interfering in its production. They're particularly effective if combined with one of the bile-acid binding resins, reducing cholesterol by 20–30 per cent and increasing HDL by a similar margin.

The snag is that such large doses of this vitamin cause unpleasant side-effects, especially itching, flushing and rashes. Two clones are commonly prescribed – nicofuranose and acipimox – each of which has far fewer side-effects.

Probucol

This drug lowers cholesterol by an unknown mechanism, perhaps as an anti-oxidant. Unfortunately, it also reduces 'good' HDL by as much as 25 per cent. So it is not a very useful therapy.

HMG CoA enzyme inhibitors (statins)

These new medications work by inhibiting an enzyme called HMG CoA reductase, which is involved in the synthesis of cholesterol by every cell of the body. The cells are forced to glean their cholesterol from the bloodstream, thus lowering the level. A reduction of up to 45 per cent has been reported, making these drugs the most effective treatment available to date.

The most widely prescribed members of this group are

simvastatin and pravastatin. They have few known side-effects, but, because they're so new, we have no idea what they do to people taking them for decades. They are also enormously expensive.

All the medications mentioned above have to be prescribed, either by a doctor or the specialist at the lipid clinic. They may sometimes be used in combination with each other, and always together with a cholesterol-lowering diet and exercise programme.

– 8 –
Eating for Life

The good news is that the balance of foods we are recommended to eat to lower our cholesterol and give our hearts a new start is the diet that will also help to keep us slim and protect us against a number of chronic diseases, including cancer. It's a diet for all-round health. It's literally eating for life.

Even better news is that it can be truly delicious.

Prehistoric fare

This healthy diet corresponds very closely to what we know about what our prehistoric ancestors consumed. The food eaten by the hunter-gatherers of the Great Rift Valley in Africa came largely from plant sources – fruits, roots and shoots – with occasional meat or fish. Grains and pulses became increasingly present as cultivation and agriculture developed. For most early humans, the only salt available was what was naturally present in these foods, and the only sugar came from fruit and vegetables. It was a diet very low in saturated fats and very high in fibre-rich starchy foods. Everything was fresh, seasonal and natural.

Today's convenience food

Our bodies are almost identical to those of our ancient forebears, but many of us live in very different circumstances, in modern developed societies, and our day-to-day diet is a far cry from the one that shaped our evolution.

The typical modern Western diet consists largely of highly processed foods – refined, emulsified, expanded, stabilised, preserved – and much of the natural balance of nutrients has been disturbed. In our relatively affluent society we can afford more meat and dairy 'luxuries' – and we're less inclined to bulk out our meals with starchy staples like potatoes, rice or pasta, or chew our way through heaps of beans or leafy vegetables.

Convenience is what matters for most of us – the fast fry-up, the pot snack or the microwave meal-in-a-minute.

Clear guidelines

Experts throughout the world have come to the conclusion that the average Western diet is far too high in saturated fat, and far too low in fibre-rich starchy foods – and that we're also eating too much salt and sugar.

Many national and international committees have drawn up clear recommendations as to how our diets should be balanced. All these committees (more than 60 of them!) agree on the main messages. Despite stories that keep appearing in the media about new findings that over-turn traditional dietary advice, scientists changing their minds or this or that food being good for you after all, the guidelines for a healthy diet are still essentially the same as they were over 15 years ago.

The most far-reaching guidelines have recently been set out by the World Health Organization in its international report, 'Diet, Nutrition and the Prevention of Chronic Diseases'. Following them will help you lower your cho-lesterol and stay slim. They'll also help to protect you from premature heart disease, strokes and some forms of cancer. What's more, the guidelines fully endorse some of the world's most delicious cuisines.

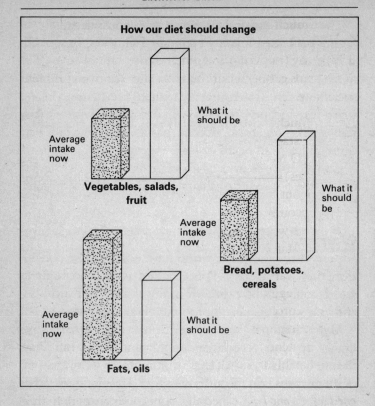

How our diet should change

How our diet must change

In the simplest of terms, the main aims for most of us in changing to a healthier balance of foods are to:

✳ eat less fat, especially saturated fat

✳ eat more fibre

✳ eat less salt

✳ eat sugar less often

But these aims refer to food *constituents* rather than to foods themselves. So, how should we change what we actually choose to eat?

126

* **Eat much more fruit, vegetables and salads.**
The WHO recommends a *minimum* of 400 g (just under 1 lb) a day (not counting potatoes).

It means eating about *five portions* of fruit or vegetables every day.

* **Eat much more bread, potatoes, cereals, rice, lentils or other starchy foods.**
The WHO recommends that starchy foods (complex carbohydrates) should provide 50–70 per cent of our calories. That's about twice as much as they do at present in most Western countries.

It means we should *double* our intake of these and other fibre-rich starchy foods.

* **Think carefully about meat, meat products, dairy products, eggs, cooking oils and other fatty foods.**
The main problem here is fat, especially saturated fat. The WHO recommends that we derive no more than 30 per cent of our energy (calories) from fats and oils of all types, and preferably less than that (minimum 15 per cent).

This means that most of us should cut our fat intake by *one-third to one-half*, especially from foods that are high in saturated fat.

* **Consider chicken, turkey and fish as alternatives.**
Poultry meat is less fatty than most red meat, with much less saturated fat. Oily fish are fatty, but relatively low in saturated fats and high in heart-healthier omega-3 polyunsaturates. White fish contain very little fat indeed.

* **Cut down on sugary foods – sweets, cakes, biscuits, ice cream, sugary soft drinks and sugar itself.**
Refined sugar is a concentrated source of calories but has no other significant nutrient value. So, cutting down on sugary foods will help you to control your weight and still eat the recommended proportion of healthier alternatives,

like starchy foods. Fewer sugary snacks and drinks will also help to prevent tooth decay.

The WHO says we have no need whatsoever for refined sugar, and recommends that a *maximum* of 10 per cent of our calorie intake is in this form.

For most people, this means that they must cut their consumption of sugar (in all the sugary foods mentioned above) by *about half*.

The chances are that you're well aware of what constitutes a healthy diet in broad terms like these. Surveys show that most people know they should eat less fat, sugar and salt and more fibre. The basic messages are also getting through to food manufacturers – many healthier alternatives are now available on supermarket shelves.

But three commonly held beliefs seem to prevent many people from taking advantage of their knowledge about healthy eating and the choice that's available. They think it's too boring, too fiddly, or too expensive.

Wrong, wrong, wrong!

Some of the most enticing and delicious cuisines in the world are also among the healthiest. Traditional Mediterranean food, for instance, with its emphasis on fresh, lightly cooked vegetables, or salads, together with bread, pasta or rice, abundant fish and a little meat, topped with aromatic herbs and rounded off with the freshest of fruits. Or the food of the Indian subcontinent, largely based on rice and vegetables, with its amazing range of exotic and scintillating spices. Or Oriental food, again rice-based or with oodles of noodles plus lots of fresh vegetables (stir-fried very quickly), chicken, duck or, certainly in Japan, fish galore.

Nor need healthy eating be fiddly. Reaching for an apple, or opening a carton of low-fat yoghurt, isn't too troublesome. Cutting a thick slice of wholemeal bread, or heating some baked beans, needn't take too much effort. Preparing a healthy salad takes a mere trice. Steaming fish or leafy vegetables takes only a little longer. And if you have a freezer and a microwave, you can make your own 'convenience' meals for the week in one session.

Finally, a healthy diet needn't break your budget. The cost depends entirely on what foods you choose. Sirloin steak is expensive – but chicken isn't. Salmon is a luxury – but sardines are a real bargain. Vegetables and fruit, in season, are excellent value – and even cheaper at a market stall. Frozen vegetables cost a little more than fresh ones, but that's the price of convenience. Staples like wholemeal bread, potatoes, cereals, wholegrain rice, yams and cassava are all relatively cheap. On the other hand, carry-outs and pre-cooked microwave dinners usually are not – and if you have them often, can really push the family food bill up.

Choosing a healthier balance

Let's assume you've decided to change your, or your family's, diet to make it healthier and more likely to help keep cholesterol levels down. How do you go about it?

It depends on whether you're a revolutionary or a 'softly-softly' person. Revolutionaries go for the grand slam. They completely transform their entire diet in one fell swoop – eating acres of fruit and vegetables, cutting red meat down or out, switching to low-fat alternatives for virtually everything (and usually taking up aerobics or jogging at the same time). 'Softly-softlies' make the odd change here and there, in gradual, easy-to-manage steps.

Either approach is fine, if it works for you. The first has the advantage that it builds on a highly motivated decision to start a new lifestyle and switch rapidly to 'the new you' – rather like being 'born again'. By making big changes all at once, you'll feel the difference that this makes, and this may reinforce your determination to stay with the changes.

On the other hand, you, or more particularly your family, may not welcome this kind of earth-shattering disruption of the day-to-day routine – and you may find yourself facing a resentful counter-revolution. So, the gradualist, softly-softly approach may be more successful in the long run. Start, perhaps, by changing to semi-skimmed milk, followed a month or so later by a switch to wholemeal bread. A while after that, introduce one or two evening meals a week without meat, and so on.

Essentials of the Mediterranean diet

The closest that European food comes to meeting the WHO guidelines for healthy eating is the typical diet in Mediterranean areas such as the south of France, southern Italy, Yugoslavia and Greece, where heart-disease rates are the lowest in Europe.

Here's how to change your diet to follow their example.

* **Very much more** fruit and vegetables

* **Much more** bread, beans, potatoes, pasta, rice, cereals

* **Much more** fish

* **Much less** fatty meat products and full-fat dairy food

* **Much less** salty food, but **many more** herbs and spices

* **Much less** frying, but **more** baking and steaming

* Use olive oil or some other highly unsaturated oil

* Drink plenty of water . . . and perhaps a little wine!

Vegetables, salads and fruit

Look round any supermarket or street market these days and you'll have to admit that the variety of fruit and vegetables on display is truly stunning. The different colours and shapes are a visual feast, and there's such a wonderful range of flavours and textures that the culinary possibilities are endless. Going Mediterranean is a delight.

All these things are good for you. Not only do they help to provide the dietary fibre you need, they also contain important vitamins and minerals. And, in the case of pulse vegetables (such as beans, peas and lentils) they make a

---

Vitamins and cholesterol

The key vitamins as far as your cholesterol is concerned are Vitamin C, Vitamin E and beta-carotene (Vitamin A). These are thought to act as anti-oxidants, scavenging or mopping up the so-called 'free radicals' produced by normal cell activity in every tissue of the body. There's increasing evidence to suggest that, in the walls of the arteries, free radicals hasten the formation of cholesterol-containing atheroma. Hence diets high in these vitamins – such as the classic Mediterranean diet – are likely to have an anti-atheroma effect, helping to protect against heart disease and strokes. Incidentally, there's evidence that these anti-oxidants also help to fight some cancers.

Vitamin C is present in a wide variety of fruit, vegetables and salads – especially most citrus fruits, blackcurrants, guavas, broccoli, beet, greens, parsley and peppers. It is partly destroyed by cooking and fine chopping.

Beta-carotene is also present in many plant foods – especially carrots, spinach, sweet potatoes, watercress, apricots, broccoli, mangoes, sweet melons, red peppers and lettuce. It is not destroyed by cooking.

Vitamin E is plentiful in various plant and animal foods. Wheatgerm and oatmeal are good sources, and it's also present in most plant oils and many green leafy vegetables. Like beta-carotene, it is not destroyed by cooking.

---

substantial contribution to your protein and complex carbohydrate (starch) intake.

Needless to say, vegetables, salads and fruit contain virtually no fat or oil (apart from the oils – mostly unsaturated – in seeds, nuts and avocado pears). No food of plant origin contains cholesterol itself.

Plan on each member of the family having at least five portions of vegetables, fruit or salad every day. This does not include potatoes, which we'll deal with separately. It does, however, include nuts – but avoid the salted variety.

Fresh, tinned or frozen?

For best value in fresh greengroceries, it makes sense to choose local produce that's in season – in winter, you'll have to pay extra for imported varieties. Some air-freighted exotic fruits, such as mangoes, papayas and guavas, although rather expensive, are delicious treats.

Tinned fruit and vegetables retain much of their goodness – in particular, fibre, Vitamin E and beta-carotene are preserved – but Vitamin C is largely lost in the canning process. Another problem with tinned foods is the frequent addition of sugar to the syrup of some fruit, and salt to some vegetables. Read the labels carefully, and look for foods canned in natural juice or labelled low sugar or salt.

Quick-frozen vegetables and fruit are much less likely to lose Vitamin C, providing you don't keep them in the freezer for too long.

Cooking vegetables

Speed is of the essence – the longer vegetables are hot, the more Vitamin C is lost. Steaming in just a little water helps because the Vitamin C isn't washed away. It's also much better than boiling for retaining the flavour, colour and goodness of the vegetable. Steamers are available in good kitchen shops – but a colander in a saucepan does the trick.

Stir-frying is another quick method of cooking vegetables, and uses a tiny amount of oil. For this, you really need a wok (again from good kitchen shops). You'll have to dice the vegetables into small pieces so that they all cook at the same speed.

Best of all, try to eat as many vegetables as possible raw in salads.

Salads

With a little effort you can make a salad that looks and tastes truly wonderful – gone are the dreary days of limp lettuce and tired cucumber.

Almost any vegetable, fruit or nut can be used (and, if you're feeling adventurous, quite a few other plants such as young dandelion leaves, chickweed, fat-hen and nasturtium flowers). Celery, apple, walnut and raisin salad is a favourite.

If you have a weight problem, go easy on oily dressings or mayonnaise. Try dressings using low-fat yoghurt and lemon juice instead.

Bread, potatoes and cereals

These are starchy foods which, along with such other staples as rice, pasta, sweetcorn (maize), noodles, cassava (tapioca), sago, plantain, sweet potato and yam, are the basis of virtually every diet throughout the world. Apart from the energy they provide from complex carbohydrates (starch), they are also important sources of fibre, vitamins (especially B vitamins in the grains, and Vitamin C in potatoes) and minerals. The WHO recommends that we double our intake of these starchy staples.

The Mediterranean diet, with its cornucopia of bread, potatoes, pasta or rice, is well-stocked with healthy starch.

Are they fattening?

Slimmers have been worrying themselves for decades that foods like bread and potatoes are fattening.

In fact, all of the starchy staples have a *low* calorie-density – and weight for weight they're less fattening than protein! What's more, because they're so filling, giving your meals satisfying bulk, you'll have less room to over-indulge in them. So, unlike sugary, fatty or high-protein foods, starchy foods have their own built-in appetite-suppressant. Indeed, recent evidence from the United States suggests that too little starchy food causes the body's metabolism to adopt a 'starvation mode', and lay down body fat as a defence.

The wrong kind of dieting can make you fat!

Pulses

Pulses need special mention with regard to preparation and cooking. They are dried beans, peas and lentils and are excellent sources of complex carbohydrates, fibre (especially the soluble, cholesterol-lowering type) protein, vitamins and minerals. What's more, they contain virtually no fat at all. They are traditional Greek, Middle Eastern and Indian fare, but are currently enjoying a real boom among Western nations. They are also very good value and, because they are dried, can be stored indefinitely.

The main disadvantage is that they need pre-soaking in three times their volume of water for at least 5 hours (except lentils, which don't need to be soaked at all). The water should then be thrown away, because it may contain natural substances which can cause wind or colic.

Cooking times, at a gentle simmer, vary from pulse to pulse – but it's important to give all of them a 10-minute fast boil to start with, to destroy any remaining colic-causing substances. This applies especially to red kidney beans. If you're pressure-cooking pulses, you don't need to fast-boil them first because the heat is high enough anyway.

The calorie-density is even lower if you choose 'whole' versions of the grain foods – wholemeal bread, wholewheat pasta, brown rice and other whole cereals – which contain more calorie-free fibre.

Needless to say, if you're concerned about calories you have to watch what you're spreading on your bread, cooking your potatoes in, or putting on your cereals.

About bread
Doctors and nutritionists are now recognising the true value of bread – not only as a source of starch and fibre, but also of protein, vitamins and minerals.

But breads differ considerably in appearance, taste, texture and nutritional content.

Pulse	*Simmering time*
Aduki beans	45 minutes
Black beans	1 hour
Black-eyed beans	1 hour
Borlotti beans	1 hour
Broad beans	1½ hours
Butter beans	1 hour
Cannelini beans	1 hour
Chick peas	1–1½ hours
Flageolet beans	1 hour
Haricot beans	1 hour
Lentils (split)	30 minutes
Lima beans	1 hour
Mung beans	30 minutes
Pinto beans	1 hour
Red kidney beans	1 hour
Soya beans	3 hours
Split peas	1 hour

Wholemeal bread is made from the whole of the wheat grain, including the wheatgerm (embryo) and the outer fibrous husk (bran). Wheatgerm is a good source of protein and the anti-oxidant Vitamin E (see page 131). Bran is an excellent source of fibre. Wholemeal bread is tastier, chewier and lower in calories than other breads. Fibre content: 8.5 per cent.

Brown bread has had about half its bran and wheatgerm stripped away in the mill. It comes in different varieties: some with added caramel to colour them, some with peahusks to increase the fibre content and some with added wheatgerm to increase protein. Vitamin B, calcium and iron are added to replace that lost in milling. A plain brown loaf has a fibre content of 5.1 per cent.

White bread has lost nearly all its bran and wheatgerm in milling. Nevertheless, it still contains useful amounts of fibre and protein. As with brown bread, Vitamin B, calcium and iron are added to make up the losses. Other additives give it a soft, springy feel and longer shelf-life. Fibre content: 2.7 per cent.

One problem with nearly all breads is that they contain rather a lot of salt – perhaps a problem for your blood pressure. However, you can compensate for this to some extent by not adding salt to whatever you're eating with the bread. If you have to be especially strict, try baking your own bread with wholemeal flour, using a little less salt each time. Although bread without salt at first tastes bland to most people, you'll soon get used to the taste.

Another problem is the amount, and type, of fat you spread on bread. We look at this more closely on page 146. But, from what we've said already, it's clear that the thicker the slice of bread you cut, the more goodness you put under each smear of spread. Doorsteps – especially wholemeal – are in!

If you haven't done so already – discover real sandwiches. Unlike the curly white variety with barely discernible fillings, real sandwiches are made with chunky wholemeal bread crammed with scrumptious low-fat or high polyunsaturate fillings: low-fat cheese and apple, low-fat coleslaw and chicken, tuna and avocado, and many others.

About potatoes

What a great vegetable is the humble spud – especially in its skin. Much of the fibre (especially the soluble, cholesterol-lowering type) and most of the Vitamin C is in, or just under, the skin. So, whenever possible, cook and eat potatoes whole – in their jackets. Instead of peeling them, simply scrub them clean.

Keep potatoes in a cool, dark place to preserve their Vitamin C and freshness.

One of the best ways of cooking them is dry-baking in an earthenware, lidded pot in the oven, so that they cook in their own moisture. Alternatively, wrap each potato in foil and bake on an open tray.

You can make delicious low-fat, or high-polyunsaturate fillings for your baked potatoes: cottage cheese and chives, chopped ham and baked beans, tuna and onion, sardine and tomato.

Even chips can be healthier if you cut them thicker, use a high-polyunsaturate oil, and keep the oil very hot.

About cereals

Like fruit and vegetables, wholegrain breakfast cereals are compulsory low-fat eating if you want to keep cholesterol down. But you have to read the packets carefully – they vary enormously in their fibre, sugar and salt content.

In general, those labelled 'wholegrain', 'wholewheat', 'all bran', 'high bran', 'added bran' or 'high in fibre' are the ones to choose. In general, the more fibre, the fewer calories per serving. Some cereals are very low in fibre – rice crispies, for example, have only one-twentieth of the amount in bran flakes.

Muesli, with its munchable mixture of oats, cereal flakes, nuts and dried fruit, is obviously a good source of fibre, and also of protein, vitamins and minerals. The nuts provide essential polyunsaturates.

Since the recent upsurge of interest in oatbran as a rich source of cholesterol-lowering soluble fibre (see page 68), many more oatbran-containing cereals have appeared on the supermarket shelves. Again, read the nutritional information on the packet to compare proportions of fibre (especially soluble fibre, if separately labelled), sugar and salt.

You do have to keep an eye on sugar content, not only with packeted cereals – some are nearly half sugar! – but also with muesli mixtures, which may have a surprising amount of added sugar – brown or white, it's just as fattening. Look for 'low sugar' or 'no added sugar' versions.

On the subject of salt, again check carefully. Some high-bran cereals are loaded with the stuff – whereas puffed and shredded wheat are relatively low in salt.

Any time is breakfast time with a bowl of cereal. Add chopped banana, pear or apple, or scatter segments of tangerine or satsuma, to give it extra zest and goodness. And, of course, the milk you add should be skimmed or semi-skimmed.

Meat, fish, dairy products and eggs

These foods are particularly crucial as far as your, and your family's, cholesterol is concerned. Apart from cooking fats and oils, they are the main sources of saturated fat and cholesterol in the diet. But they're also highly nutritious and flavoursome, and do much to make eating a delight. So, with all these foods, the message is to enjoy them in moderation and balance, with the emphasis on lower fat and higher polyunsaturate alternatives.

Meat

Take red meat, for example. People often think that it is high in fat and therefore can't be healthy. But that's forgetting two important points.

Firstly, there are several ways of reducing meat's fat contribution:

* Choose leaner cuts

* Cut off visible fat

* Grill or bake rather than fry

* Skim the fat from stews and casseroles

* Replace some of the meat with vegetables or pulses.

Secondly, meat is a good source of other nutrients like protein, iron, zinc and vitamins (all the B vitamins and Vitamin A). So, red meat, although certainly not an essential food, can be part of a healthy cholesterol-lowering diet provided it's used in the right way.

In general, though, nearly half the fat in meat and meat products is saturated – the kind that pushes up blood cholesterol. All in all, these foods contribute about a quarter of the saturated-fat content of the average Western diet. If you eat meat, it's important to choose carefully, remove as much fat as possible when you cook it, and enjoy it in moderation.

In most Mediterranean dishes the meat, if any, is frequently grilled and balanced with plenty of delicious vegetables.

Fat content of raw meats

Meat	Type	Total fat content (%)
Beef	lean average	5
	sirloin (lean + fat)	23
Lamb	lean average	9
	leg (lean + fat)	19
Pork	lean average	4
	leg (lean + fat)	13
Chicken	meat only	4
	meat + skin	18
Offal	pig's liver	3
	lamb's kidney	3
Bacon	lean average	4
	streaky	24
	gammon	13

Note: These are *raw* meats. Some fat is lost in cooking – more so in grilling or baking than in frying.

Most meat products like sausages, pies, pasties and pâtés have a very high fat content. Some, notably salami, sausage rolls, pork pies, liver sausage and pâté, contain much more fat than most raw meats.

What about offal?

Broadly speaking, liver, kidneys and heart are about half as fatty as other meat from the same animal. But offal does contain quite a lot of dietary cholesterol – about four to six times as much as the meat. Brain is brimming with the stuff, and kidneys are also crammed with it. There's lots in liver. If your cholesterol level is high, be sure to go very easy on offal.

Nevertheless, as we saw in Chapter 2, the cholesterol we eat contributes only a small proportion of the cholesterol in our bloodstream. Far and away the largest factor raising blood cholesterol is the fat content of our food, especially the saturated fat.

Milk and dairy foods

Milk, cheese and cream are other major sources of fat in our food and drink, supplying nearly one-fifth of the average person's fat intake. If you include butter, the gentle cow is clearly our leading supplier of fat, particularly saturated fat.

Over two-thirds of the fat in milk, butter, cheese and cream is saturated, and all in all these foods are the source of about 40 per cent of the saturated fat we consume. Clearly, we have to choose our dairy products with care.

And yet they are also an important source of many vital nutrients, including protein, calcium (for strong teeth and bones) and Vitamins A, B complex, C, D, E and folic acid.

Fortunately, we now have a variety of low-fat milks, yoghurts, cheeses and 'creams' available, which retain their protein and calcium content. However, because Vitamins A, D and E in particular are removed with the fat, these products are not suitable for children under five, who should be given whole milk instead.

The fat in dairy products

Product	Total fat (%)	Saturated fat (%)
Whole milks		
Channel Islands (gold top)	4.9	3.1
(silver-top or homogenised)	3.9	2.5
Semi-skimmed milk		
(red stripes)	1.6	1.0
Skimmed milk (blue check)	.1	.06

Product	Total fat (%)	Saturated fat (%)
Double cream	48.0	30.7
Whipping cream	35.0	22.4
Single cream	19.0	12.2
Half cream	12.3	7.9
Ice cream (dairy vanilla)	9.8	6.4
Greek yoghurt (cow's milk)	9.1	5.2
Plain yoghurt	3.0	1.7
Plain low-fat yoghurt	.8	.5
Plain very low-fat yoghurt	.1	.06
Butter	81.0	51.8
Cream cheese	47.4	30.3
Stilton	35.0	22.4
Cheddar	34.4	22.0
Double Gloucester	34.0	21.7
Gruyère	32.0	20.5
Wensleydale	31.5	20.2
Cheshire	31.4	20.1
Caerphilly	31.3	20.0
Danish Blue	29.2	18.7
Emmental	29.0	18.6
Gouda	28.2	18.1
Gorgonzola	26.4	16.9
Camembert	23.2	14.8
Brie	23.0	14.7
Edam	22.9	14.6
Half-fat Cheddar	16.5	10.5
Low-fat soft cheese	8.6	5.5
Fromage frais	6.6	4.2
Cottage cheese	4.1	2.6
Low-fat cottage cheese	1.8	1.1

Going fishing

As we saw in Chapter 5, there's renewed interest in fish as an important source of 'long-chain omega-3' polyunsaturates, which seem to have a double protective effect against heart disease. They not only help to increase the level of HDL, the beneficial blood lipid, but also reduce the tendency of the blood to form clots – an anti-thrombosis effect.

Oily fish contain far more of these long-chain omega-3 polyunsaturates than white fish – but fish oil, like any other oil, is highly calorific. So, you seem to be faced with a choice: to go for heart protection or to watch your weight.

In practice, of course, you can do both, by making room for the extra calories in oily fish. In other words, replace one or two meat- or cheese-based meals each week with the equivalent calories in oily fish. If you need actually to lose calories, swap another meat meal or two for one or two based on white fish, which has very little oil and about half the calories of oily fish.

The choice of fish is enormous. Fresh, frozen or tinned fish are best for healthy eating – smoked or brine-pickled fish are tasty treats, but very salty.

The main oily fish in countries like Britain are:

* herring

* mackerel

* sardine

* salmon

* tuna

* pilchard

* whiting

* eel

And here are some of the best ways to cook fish for a healthy diet. Remember, it cooks very quickly. Don't overdo it.

✱ **Grilling and barbecuing.** Some of the oil is lost, but you can baste with lemon juice and dill.

✱ **Poaching.** Simmer in skimmed milk or stock, and use the liquor as a sauce. Delicious!

✱ **Steaming.** In a steamer or fish kettle or in a colander with a lid.

✱ **Baking.** Wrap the fish in foil. Even tastier with herb stuffing.

✱ **Stir-frying.** Small cubes of fish cook really quickly this way. Just a little polyunsaturated oil and add some chopped vegetables.

✱ **Microwaving.** A little lemon juice helps to keep the fish moist. Whole fish need slitting to prevent bursting. Keep covered.

If you have to fry your fish, use a polyunsaturated oil and drain it before you serve. Needless to say, fish in batter is loaded with calories. More important as far as your cholesterol is concerned, most fish-and-chip shops use blended vegetable oil for frying – highly saturated.

Shellfish
Wonderfully enticing, shellfish add something really special to a meal. From the ubiquitous prawn to the occasional oyster, and from the humble mussel to the revered lobster – not to mention crabs, scampi, squid, cockles, shrimps, whelks, crayfish and winkles – they're all wonderful. And they're all low in fat.

Some shellfish – particularly shrimps and prawns – contain quite high levels of dietary cholesterol. But it amounts to a tiny proportion of the total cholesterol in your food and, providing you don't go overboard on these delights, is frankly not worth worrying about.

Chicken, turkey and duck

Not only are chicken and turkey excellent value, but they're also low in fat. What's more, the fat they do contain is mostly in the skin and (if you're watching your weight) can easily be removed. Incidentally, it is mostly unsaturated – mono and poly – and therefore healthier for the heart than the fat in red meat.

Duck is much richer in fat than chicken or turkey. Again, it is mostly just under the skin, but in a much thicker layer. The fat is three-quarters unsaturated, and very oily, giving the duck meat a delicious flavour. Apart from the calories, it's relatively 'healthy' fat – but, because it's so rich, it does need a fruity sauce such as orange or cherry.

Eggs

Which came first in the cholesterol story, the chicken or the egg?

Long before chicken became a cheaper and healthier alternative to red meat, the egg was branded as the enemy of the people because of its high dietary cholesterol content. There's no denying that yolks do contain more than their fair share of cholesterol – about 10 times as much as double cream. But even so, it amounts to only just over 1 per cent of each yolk – the rest is sheer goodness. There's no cholesterol in egg whites.

If you have a high blood cholesterol, it's sensible to restrict your egg consumption to no more than two or three per week. The WHO recommendation for the general population is up to four a week on average. But don't forget, this includes the eggs used in cake mixes and pastries.

Fats and oils

We come at last to the big one – fats and oils – the foods that supply more of the fat we eat than any other group. More than meat and meat products. More than milk, cheese and cream. And much more than poultry, fish and all the rest. The way we use fats and oils has more bearing on our blood cholesterol than anything else in our diet. It can also have a sizeable effect on our waistlines.

Fats and oils include butter and margarines, low-fat spreads, cooking oils, lard and suet.

As far as calories are concerned, the oils are a little more fattening than the fats because the latter contain water – lard about 1 per cent, butter/margarines about 15 per cent.

But in terms of saturated fat, the hard fats are the main culprits – although not entirely.

Here's how fats and oils are divided according to which type of fatty-acid constituent is predominant. They are in descending order: the items at the top of each column have the highest proportion of that particular type of fatty acid, those at the bottom have the lowest.

Mainly saturated	*Mainly monounsaturated*	*Mainly polyunsaturated*
Palm kernel oil	Olive oil	Safflower oil
Coconut oil	Rapeseed oil	Sunflower oil
Butter	Groundnut oil	Polyunsaturated
Palm oil	Beef dripping	margarines
Lard	Corn (maize) oil	Soya oil
Suet	Ordinary soft	Walnut oil
	margarines	
	Hard margarines	

To keep your cholesterol down, therefore, you should try to substitute items in the saturated column with equivalents as close as possible to the top of the monounsaturated or polyunsaturated columns.

Each oil has its own special flavour, which may not be suitable for all dishes you prepare, so experiment a little. Also, some oils – olive oil and walnut oil, for example – are much more expensive than others like corn oil and groundnut oil.

To convert a recipe calling for butter or hard margarine into one using oil, remember that 4 oz (100 g) of the former is equivalent to 5 tablespoons (75 ml) of the latter.

Low-fat spreads are not suitable for frying or baking because they contain a large amount of water. They have about half the fat of butter or margarine, and only two-thirds of the saturated fat in polyunsaturated margarine. They are also low in unsaturated fats. Very low-fat spreads contain even more water and have about the same proportion of fat as processed cheese (25 per cent).

Seasonings
Low-fat food needn't be dull. There are lots of ways of bringing meals to life without adding either fat or calories.

Salt
Use it sparingly – too much is linked to high blood pressure. Sea-salt tastes nicer, but contains virtually the same amount of sodium. Wean yourself slowly off salt. There's no need to cut it out altogether, but use much less than usual in cooking and at the table. Salt substitutes which contain more potassium than sodium are available – but they may not be suitable if you already have heart or kidney trouble. Half the salt we eat is added to food during manufacture. Stock cubes are about one-quarter salt!

Pepper

An excellent way of perking up the taste-buds without the drawbacks of salt. Black pepper is much more aromatic and not just peppery. Use it freshly ground with a peppermill.

Herbs

Basil   In vegetable soups; tomato soup; beef stew; fish; sprinkled on fresh tomatoes, aubergine, asparagus and broccoli.

Bay leaves   In soups and stews.

Caraway   With pork, coleslaw, cabbage, turnips, rye and pumpernickel bread.

Chives   With cabbage, potatoes, courgettes, omelettes.

Dill   As garnish on fish, potato salad, sliced cucumber; with beans, cabbage, cauliflower, potatoes.

Fennel   With fish; with sliced tomato, onion; in bread.

Garlic   In salads and many savoury dishes. Thought to have cholesterol-lowering properties (see page 70).

Marjoram   In soups, stews; with grilled or baked fish; with chicken, veal, lamb; in scones.

Mint   With lamb; in pea soup; in salads; in fruit drinks.

Oregano   In tomato juice or soups; meat sauces; meat balls; pizzas.

Parsley   As garnish on savouries; meats; fish.

Rosemary   In chicken, spinach or pea soup; on chicken, lamb or veal; in baked fish; in salad dressings; potato salad.

Sage   In consommé or yoghurt soups; on poultry or pork; with beans.

Tarragon   In salad dressings, sauces; with fish, chicken and savouries.

Thyme   In soups; with fish; in dumplings.

Spices

Allspice   With tomato and pea soups; in roasts or marinades; in poached fish; on fruit salad; in salad dressings.

Cinnamon On lean lamb chops; in stews; on tomatoes; on cottage cheese; over oranges, bananas, berries and apples.

Cloves In borscht, split pea, potato soup; with baked fish; ground and sprinkled over beans, cucumber, tomatoes; in apple and pear desserts.

Ginger On chicken; on pears; on beetroot, carrots, cucumber; in fruit salad.

Mace In casseroles; in sauces for vegetables.

Mustard With casseroles, meat loaves, hamburgers, sausages or roast beef.

Nutmeg With chicken soup; in meat loaf; on chicken; in fishcakes; on carrots, beans, spinach, peas; in fruit salad; on custard.

Paprika As garnish in soups and on raw vegetables; on chicken and veal; on fish; on yoghurt-covered vegetables.

Shopping for a healthy heart

We're now in a position to go shopping for the foods we need for healthy, low-fat eating and drinking. Remember the key words: variety and balance. Look again at page 127 for the basic WHO recommendations. These give the basic themes for your shopping list. To summarise:

✳ Lots more vegetables, salads and fruit. No limit. The fresher, the better.

✳ At least double the amount of bread, potatoes, cereals, rice, pasta and other staples. Whole is best.

✳ Cut right down on fat. A conscious effort to buy about half as much fatty food as we do at present is likely to result in the reduction the WHO recommends. But, faced with the choice, give preference to foods higher in unsaturated fats. Remember what we've said about meat, dairy foods, poultry, eggs, fish and fats and oils.

✳ You know this one well enough! Go easy on sweets, chocolate, cakes, biscuits and other sugary or fatty treats. For the occasional indulgence only.

✳ Soft-pedal on the drink. Remember the advice about alcohol on page 111.

Your shopping basket
Armed with these basic principles, let's start filling up the shopping basket with some healthier alternatives.

Fruit and vegetables
Linger a long time in the greengrocery section in your supermarket. Here, you could fill your whole basket with luscious delights. Choose a selection of fresh fruit (including lemons), potatoes, greens, carrots and salad vegetables – whatever takes your fancy. Move on and stock up with frozen vegetables too – peas, beans, broccoli and low-fat oven chips (probably unavoidable!). At the tinned shelf: baked beans, sweetcorn, red kidney beans, chick peas, tomatoes. Look for vegetables without added salt, and fruit in natural juice. Choose unsweetened fruit juices.

Dairy foods, fats and oils, cooked meats
Choose semi-skimmed or skimmed milk (but whole milk for under-fives). Plain or fruit low-fat yoghurts (or very low fat), and low-fat fromage frais. Lower-fat cheeses. Polyunsaturated margarine (preferably pure sunflower) and low-fat spread (you'll need both, for cooking and spreading). Eggs (use sparingly). Pure safflower or sunflower oil (or a cheaper high-polyunsaturated alternative). Pure olive oil (or a cheaper high-monounsaturated alternative). Lean ham. Low-fat sausages.

Fresh and frozen meat
Lean cuts, lean mince. Chicken or chicken pieces, turkey. Low-fat burgers.

Fresh, frozen and tinned fish
Any fish – white or oily. Steady with the roes (very high in cholesterol). Shellfish galore. Frozen fish (yes, even fish fingers!). Tinned tuna, sardines, pilchards, salmon. Anchovies for seasoning only (very salty).

Other foods
Wholemeal flour for breadmaking and pastries. Baker's yeast. Cornflour or arrowroot for thickening. Rolled oats and oatbran (for muesli and muffins). Wholegrain breakfast cereals (branflakes, wheatbisks, puffed wheat). Brown rice. Wholewheat pasta. Wholemeal bread, rolls, pitta. Wholegrain crispbread. Dried fruits (raisins, apricots, bananas). Nuts. Dried pulses (a variety of beans, peas and lentils). Herbs and spices.

You can get virtually all these things in a supermarket – as long as you read the labels carefully. But it's more interesting to shop around. There's usually a larger choice in your high street butcher, baker, greengrocer and fishmonger – or, for keener prices, at the street market. And don't forget your local wholefood store, for a wider choice of pulses, grains, nuts, dried fruits and pasta.

Low-fat cooking
There's no room to go into detail here, but the general principles are these:

✳ Whenever possible, eat fruit and vegetables raw or only lightly cooked. Wash thoroughly to remove pesticide residues, and dry with tissue or in a salad-spinner.

✳ Grill or bake rather than fry. Grill under a gas or electric grill, or over a charcoal barbecue. Ideal for kebabs, lean steaks and oily fish. Bake fish in foil or greaseproof paper parcels – *en papillote*.

✳ If you need to fry, use unsaturated oil or dry-fry in a coated pan. Stir-frying in a wok, using very little oil, is an excellent and fast way to cook small chunks of meat, fish, shellfish and vegetables.

✳ Deep-frying (for food like chips) can be done in a way that minimises the fat content: cut bigger pieces so that there is less surface for more volume, and use hotter oil to seal the food before it can soak up too much fat. But not so hot that the oil smokes – danger: fire!

✳ Roast meat on a rack over the roasting-tin so that the fat is separated from the joint, and can be poured off. Use a little polyunsaturated oil for roasting vegetables.

✳ Pot-roasting, braising and stewing. Skim off the fat that rises to the surface. Or cook the dish the day before and lift off the hardened fat layer that will form overnight in the refrigerator.

✳ Boiling, poaching and steaming. Good low-fat ways of cooking – but use a minimum of water and a minimum of time. Poaching or steaming is best for fish, especially white fish. Steaming leafy vegetables preserves their colour, flavour and bite.

✳ A microwave cooks fast, from the inside outwards – excellent for preserving nutrients and flavour. Particularly good for potatoes, vegetables and fruit. A jacket potato, for instance, is ready in just 4 minutes!

Snacks and treats

Life isn't worth living without snacks and treats – especially for children of all ages! Some of the healthiest nibbles are also the nicest: apples, tangerines or satsumas, bananas and unsalted nuts. And less obvious are crunchy salad things like celery, carrots, cherry tomatoes and peppers. Dried fruit, raisins and dates are good and not too sweet. Low-sugar muesli with low-fat milk is a filling snack any time. And you can bake mixed seed, nut, fruit and honey biscuits for teatime. Wonderful!

Useful Addresses

Alcohol Concern
305 Grays Inn Road, London WC1X 8QF
Tel. 071 833 3471

ASH (Action on Smoking and Health)
5–11 Mortimer Street, London W1N 7RN
Tel. 071 637 9843

British Dietetic Association
7th Floor, Elizabeth House, 22 Suffolk Street, Queensway,
Birmingham B1 1LS
Tel. 021 643 5483

British Heart Foundation
14 Fitzhardinge Street, London W1H 4DH
Tel. 071 935 0185

Chest, Heart and Stroke Association
CHSA House, Whitecross Street, London EC1Y 8JJ
Tel. 071 490 7999

Coronary Prevention Group
102 Gloucester Place, London W1H 3DA
Tel. 071 935 2889

Family Heart Association
Wesley House, 7 High Street, Kidlington, Oxford OX5 2DH
Tel 08675 70292

Food Sense
(*for Ministry of Agriculture, Fisheries and Food publications*)
Food Sense, London SE99 7TT

Health Education Authority
Hamilton House, Mabledon Place, London WC1H 9TX
Tel. 071 383 3833

Health Education Board for Scotland
Woodburn House, Canaan Lane, Edinburgh EH10 4SG
Tel. 031 447 8044

Health Promotion Agency for Northern Ireland
The Beeches, 12 Hampton Manor Drive, Belfast BT7 3EN
Tel. 0232 644811

Health Promotion Authority for Wales
8th Floor, Brunel House, 2 Fitzalan Road, Cardiff CF2 1EB
Tel. 0222 472472

HMSO Publications
(*See your local yellow pages*)

Scottish Sports Council
Caledonian House, South Gyle, Edinburgh EH12 9DQ
Tel. 031 317 7200

Sports Council
16 Upper Woburn Place, London WC1H 0QP
Tel. 071 388 1277

Sports Council for Northern Ireland
The House of Sport, Upper Malone Road, Belfast BT9 5LA
Tel. 0232 381222

Sports Council for Wales
National Sports Centre for Wales, Sophia Gardens, Cardiff
CF1 9SW
Tel. 0222 397571

Index

Other health titles available from BBC Books:

THE NEW BBC DIET
Dr Barry Lynch

FIGHT CANCER
Professor Karol Sikora and Dr Hilary Thomas

OK2
Dr Jenny Cozens